THE HISTORICAL RELATIONS

OF

MEDICINE AND SURGERY

AMS PRESS
NEW YORK

" *Or, comme il est impossible de connaître parfaitement la partie, si l'on ne connaît au moins grosso modo le tout, il est impossible d'être bon chirurgien si l'on ne connaît pas les principes et les généralités les plus importantes de la médecine. D'autre part, comme il est impossible de connaître parfaitement le tout, si l'on ne connaît dans une certaine mesure chacune de ses parties, il est impossible que celui-là soit bon médecin qui ignore absolument l'art de la chirurgie.*"

HENRI DE MONDEVILLE.

THE

HISTORICAL RELATIONS

OF

MEDICINE AND SURGERY

TO THE END OF THE SIXTEENTH CENTURY

AN ADDRESS

DELIVERED AT THE ST. LOUIS CONGRESS

IN 1904

BY

T. CLIFFORD ALLBUTT, M.A., M.D.

HON. M.D. (DUBL.), HON. LL.D. (GLASGOW)
HON. D.SC. (OXF. AND VICT.), F.R.C.P., F.R.S., F.L.S., F.S.A.

REGIUS PROFESSOR OF PHYSIC IN THE UNIVERSITY OF CAMBRIDGE
FELLOW OF GONVILLE AND CAIUS COLLEGE, HON. FELLOW
ROYAL COLLEGE OF PHYSICIANS OF IRELAND, AND
OF THE NEW YORK ACADEMY OF MEDICINE

London

MACMILLAN AND CO., Limited
NEW YORK: THE MACMILLAN COMPANY

1905

ST. PHILIP'S COLLEGE LIBRARY

Library of Congress Cataloging in Publication Data

Allbutt, Thomas Clifford, Sir, 1836-1925.
    The historical relations of medicine and surgery
to the end of the sixteenth century.

    Reprint of the 1905 ed. published by Macmillan,
London.
    Includes index.
    1. Medicine—History. 2. Surgery—History.
I. Title. [DNLM: WZ40 A421h 1905a]
R131.A57   1978   610'.9   75-23672
ISBN 0-404-13225-1

Reprinted from an original in the collections
of the Ohio State University Library

From the edition of 1905, London
First AMS edition published in 1978
Manufactured in the United States of America

AMS PRESS INC.
NEW YORK, N.Y.

ST. PHILIP'S COLLEGE LIBRARY

TO MY

MANY GENEROUS AMERICAN FRIENDS

FRIENDS AS GENEROUS IN THEIR HOSPITALITY

TO THE STRANGER

AND THEIR APPRECIATION OF HIS DIFFIDENT SERVICE

AS IN THEIR LOVE OF LEARNING

THIS TRACT IS DEDICATED

S. Francisco, 1898.
St. Louis, 1904.

084096

PREFACE

In Inner medicine, as in all the other departments of the Congress at St. Louis, two addresses were proposed—the first to deal with the outward relations of the subject, the second with its internal problems. My colleague, Dr. Thayer, was so good as to commit to me the outward relations, as in this respect I had some materials already in hand. In recent times the relations of medicine and surgery have become so complex, and in certain directions are still so perverse, that I have preferred to deal with them at their sources, and in their earlier and simpler connexions and contrasts; that is, in ancient and medieval times. In the times of Greece and Alexandria medicine and surgery were one; to the clear eye of the Greek they could not be sundered: in medieval times on the other hand new and vaster social constructions, new and more conflicting conditions, compelled our fathers to build in their eagerness on a narrow and temporary framework.

The analytic historian lays bare the Middle Ages of Europe; he goes to the sources, he works up his descriptions, and we think we are learning something of that wonderful time until we drop *pièces justificatives* for the *Canterbury Tales,* and the drone of the lecture-room for the clarion of St. Bernard, or perchance wander into one of its minsters during the *Benedicite* or the *De profundis,* and start almost with fear to discover that their deeper and richer possession seems farther from us than ever. While we were repainting their pageants, deploring their furies, refuting their dialectics, it is suddenly revealed to us that to refute the conceptions of medieval thinkers is not to explain the origin of their ideas, and that beside their vision and their passion our hearts have grown cold and slow. To the Middle Ages we may adapt the fine thought of Burke that " dark confused uncertain images have a greater power to form the grander passions than those have which are more clear and determinate." And as to our modern civilities, have not these new islanders of the Pacific put them all on before our eyes, in a few months as it were ; and dressed them even better than we have done ! Still in our way we must on, anatomising the Middle Ages and searching for the lost key of their lyrical secret, that peradventure by dismembering the body we may reach its soul. Or is it rather by chemistry that we may extract this essence ? Is it by weighing the spirit of Ionia, the spirit of Rome, the spirit of Byzantium, the spirit of Cordova, that we shall capture the essence of Chartres, of Fulda, of Paris, of Bologna, of Florence ?   One spirit, indeed, glows through all their magic, a fire never utterly extinct, the spirit of ancient Greece—of Ionia, Athens, and Greek Italy, and so of all Italy, penetrating the alien hearts of Jew and Syrian, of Gaul and Spaniard, of Frank and Teuton, and revealing to all the wonder and beauty in common things.

As we cannot know any part of an age or people without an idea of the whole, nor take to ourselves a lesson from other times and other folk without some conception of their nature and fashion, so we cannot know modern Medicine unless we study it as a whole, in the past as well as in the present. From Greece and medieval Italy we have to bring home the lesson that our division of Medicine [1] into medicine and surgery had its root not in nature, nor even in natural artifice, but in clerical feudal and humanistic conceits.   " Quae enim in natura fundata sunt crescent et augeantur ; quae autem in opinione variantur non augentur."

If we inquire more closely how Medicine fared in the fiery youth of modern Europe, we may offer at any rate two parts of the answer : first, the iron rule of prince and prelate, wicked as individual

[1] In this essay I have written "Medicine" (with capital initial) to signify our profession as a whole ; and "medicine" (with small initial) to signify "Inner medicine," as divided from surgery and obstetrics.

rulers have been, was possible because the peoples felt instinctively the radical and universal need of the age to be that the elements of the new Europe should be welded into a stable and coherent whole. This passionate idea of unity, called now the Church, now the Empire ; here visible as the feudal tramp of the crusades, there as the tyrannous vociferations of the schools, would brook no schism, ecclesiastical social or personal.   As of every other sphere, so this spirit of domination took possession of Medicine, and therein set up the idolatry of Galen as inexorably as that of Aristotle in the sphere of philosophy. Whatever at one period were the constructive effects of this despotism, when it had outlasted its time it became as oppressive to Medicine, and to all know-ledge, as formerly it had been socially integrative.

Secondly—or indeed it is another aspect of these reflections—the soul of the Middle Ages was a collective soul ; its great works were the offspring not of individuals but of peoples.   Who built the minsters, who painted the windows and the Books of Hours, who wrote the liturgies and chansons, we know not.   As the churches, the liturgies, the manuscripts, the poetry and drama were achieve-ments not so much of persons as of congregations, so also medieval learning was for the most part the learning of inspired crowds at the heels of a rhetorician.

Thus all this medieval achievement, fervid and

beautiful as it was, could not do much for science ; nor even for the intellectual harmonies of the fine arts. As the medieval spirit was multiform and catholic, the Greek spirit on the contrary was choice and personal, and owed its being to individuals— to Ictinus and Mnesicles, Phidias and Polygnotus, Homer and Aeschylus, Plato and Aristotle, Mantegna and Donatello. The Greek was an individualising and an emancipating spirit, the medieval collective and enthralling — a genius of assemblies and associations of men. It was by strife of individuals for personal development that through much suffering Greek thought and the personal life was reawakened ; and until this emancipation scientific research and intellectual art were impossible or ineffectual. In art the finer harmonies of form and the conscious appreciations of the personal artist were not medieval but Greek ; likewise in science the spirit of individual research and the freedom of individual opinion were impossible under the oppressions and the checks of collective despotisms. In this cause of the individual against society, if Luther and Knox were triumphant Dolet and Bruno were burned, Galileo and Palissy were spared reluctantly. It is interesting to reflect however that as in Italy a sense of unity never died away, even in medieval times, so in this land the need of a compulsive uniformity was less passionately felt ;

and, until the ascent of the malignant star of Spain, a larger life was open to the sciences and to Medicine, especially in the free cities of Florence and Venice. But in France a new nation had to be forged out of conflicting and reluctant elements; and therefore till consolidation was achieved the framework of custom had to be as rigid as steel. Thus in Paris Medicine, like other energies, was far more rigidly fixed by sacerdotal scholastic and military convention than in Italy; in Paris the inflexible rule of privilege strangled all quickening in science and stiffened its professors into obsequious automatons.

To the student of Greek Medicine the separation in later times of surgery from medicine, which cut most deeply in Paris, seems as false in notion as in practice it has been pernicious. If the modern surgeon is vexed to hear that surgery is, as Galen declared, but a method of treatment, he is vexed by a truth which in the best interests of our profession he ought to welcome. That in later ages in Europe the field of surgery has been avoided by the "physician," and the field of medicine forbidden to the surgeon, and that by this unnatural schism Medicine has suffered much bane, is illustrated in history, as it is day by day in the fragmentation of our work. For example, a few weeks ago an able surgeon wrote—and so far as I read him—in no ironical mood: "Let

us realise that the cæcum in these cases is the
physician's, and the appendix the surgeon's. . . .
This would make an honourable draw of the tug-
of-war." In the next paragraph he wrote : " Those
cases which apparently do not get well after an
affected appendix has been removed have only themselves and the physician to blame . . . when the
surgeon has done his share." What a mockery
for the physician no doubt the shrewd surgeon
knew well enough. Another surgeon demurely
writes : " Here I am afraid to go on lest I should
trench upon the subject of medicine." Professor
Penzoldt more frankly laments the evil of the
factitious division of practice into medicine and surgery, and sees no compensation for its disadvantages.
How ungracious a part all this is for the surgeon,
how hollow a part for the physician, how incon-
venient, mischievous and adverse to the organisation
of our science and art it is my purpose to enforce.
How many years have we lost in such maladies as
infantile palsy, diseases of the stomach, diseases of
the pelvis, and so forth, because surgeons pretend
to be " afraid to trench upon " a large and essential
part of their own pursuit, and because physicians
have been brought up in unhandy ways.

It will not be supposed that I ignore the limits
and diversities of human faculty, for to one may be
given manual dexterity, to another sagacity of observation and inference ; nor forget the field of

Medicine is so vast that for the narrowness of man's capacity it must be divided : what I urge is that the limits should be by personal choice on natural lines, not by the survival of medieval rules, even in their own day vicious, whereby we have made an idol of this divergence, telling each physician, each surgeon, that he shall not follow the bent and growth of his own faculties and the intimate tracks of nature, but that, whatever his capacities and occasions, thus far he shall go and no farther ; in the use of his natural gifts he shall be fettered by an artificial rule.   Every wise man learns, but too soon, his own defects, his own limits, his own bents, and the natural economy which they impose upon him ; but to maintain separate Colleges to intensify schism, to separate the man who treats a disease with one remedy from the man who treats the same disease with another remedy, to distribute half of a malady to one practitioner, to another the remnant, to encourage in the surgeon a show of ignorance of one portion of a disease which he has to treat, and the pretence of taking this at second hand from another, to prescribe to the physician that he may carry a merely inferential knowledge of a disease to the utmost, but shall not occupy himself with the directest way of ascertaining its intimate nature, and perhaps the only way of curing it, is contrary to nature, art and common-sense.   Surely the hour has come to amalgamate medical institu-

tions and customs, to establish an Academy of
Medicine every member of which shall be free
to develop his faculties in whatsoever honourable
paths they may lead him, and formally to recognise
an integration which, in spite of custom, in ophthal-
mology, dermatology, gynæcology, has established
itself before our eyes. In diseases of the abdomen
shall we continue to hamper and confine the
disciples of Hippocrates, Linacre, and Harvey in the
study of the anatomy of the living disease which
is the privilege of their brethren who own allegi-
ance to Hippocrates, Paré, and Hunter ? In
cerebral surgery for instance is it not absurd for
one institution to deny, let us say, to Sir William
Gowers and Professor Ferrier a liberty which by
another institution is granted, let us say, to Professors
M'Ewen and Horsley ?

It is unnecessary to carry on this argument
into the diseases of the stomach, of the peritoneum,
of the gall-bladder, of the pancreas, and so forth,
where the surgeon, besides his peculiar advantages,
has all that liberty of inferential methods with
which alone the physician has perforce to content
himself. Does not the physician see how treacherous
is the bottom of this alliance ; how rapidly the
surgeon is not only attaining " medical " sagacity
but, every day correcting sagacity in the laboratory
of living processes, is even in security and precision
of diagnosis coming to surpass the mere physician ?

Moreover—to pass to higher considerations—the habit of dwelling rather in appearance than in realities is, as Acton said, the habit of regarding the report rather than the bullet and the echo rather than the report.   Let us take for our new Academy the Wriothesley motto : " *Ung par tout et tout par ung*."

In writing of ancient authors I have preferred familiar use to scientific orthography.   Nothing does more to make history unreal than to give men pedantic names, or names which to us seem uncouth. As Horace, Avicenna, Tintoret are of " our business and bosoms," so are Galen, Salicet, Guy ; on the other hand to write John Kaye for " Caius " would be as pedantic as to substitute Albert the Great for Albertus Magnus, or von Hohenheim for Paracelsus. In doubtful instances however it is best to prefer the less exotic forms.

In conclusion I would thank my colleague Professor Howard Marsh for his charity in perusing my proofs ; but I scarcely know how to do this as I ought without seeming to lay upon him some portion of a responsibility which I must bear alone.

T. C. A.

THE HISTORICAL RELATIONS

OF

MEDICINE AND SURGERY

It was I think in the year 1864, when I was a
novice in the Honorary Staff of the Leeds General
Infirmary, that the unsurgical division of us was
summoned in great solemnity to discuss a method
of administration of drugs by means of a needle.
This method having obtained some vogue, it behoved
those who practised "pure" medicine to decide
whether the operation were consistent with the
traditions of purity. For my part I answered that
the method had come up early, if not originally, in
St. George's Hospital, and in the hands of a House
Physician—Dr. C. Hunter; that I had accustomed
myself already to the practice, and proposed to continue it; moreover that I had recently come from
the classes of Professor Trousseau who, when his
cases demanded such treatment, did not hesitate
himself to perform paracentesis of the pleura, or
even incision of this sac, or of the pericardium. As,
for lack not of will but of skill and nerve, I did not

B

intend myself to perform even minor operations, my
heresy, as one in thought only, was indulgently
ignored, and we were set free to manipulate the
drug needle, if we felt disposed to this humble
service.   About this time, when indeed few Fellows
of the London College of Physicians would con-
descend even to a digital examination of rectum
or uterus, certain of them, concerned with the
diseases of women, began to make little operations
about the uterus; and, meeting after all with but
slight rebuke, they rode on the tide of science and
circumstance, encroaching farther and farther, until
they were discovered in the act of laparotomy;
and, rather in defiance than by conversion of the
prevailing sentiment of that Corporation, they went
on doing it.

Meanwhile the surgeons, emboldened by great
events in their mystery, wrought much evil to the
" pure " physicians; accusing them with some
asperity of dawdling with cases of ileus and the
like until the opportunity of efficient treatment had
passed away: nay, audacious murmurs arose that
such " abdominal cases " should be admitted into
the surgical wards from the first.   Then by
dexterous cures growing bolder and bolder the
surgeons went so far as to make a like demand for
cases of tuberculous peritonitis, of empyema, and
even of cerebral tumour.   As thus the surgeons
laid hands on organ after organ which hitherto had
been sacred to " pure " medicine, and indeed as the
achievements of surgery became more and more
glorious, not only the man in the street but the

man of the Hospital Committee also began to
tattle about the progress of surgery and the diminu-
tion of medicine, until it was only by the natural
sweetness of our tempers that the surgeon and the
inner mediciner kept friends.   At a dinner given on
the 30th of June last to Mr. Chamberlain, in recog-
nition of his great services to tropical medicine,
this eminent statesman said, " I have often heard
that while surgery has made gigantic progress
during the last generation, medical science has
not advanced in equal proportion "; then, while
modestly disclaiming the knowledge to " distinguish
between the respective claims of these two great
professions," he generously testified that " medical
research assisted by surgical science has thrown a
flood of light on the origin of disease, and that this
at any rate is the first step to the cure of disease."
Now Mr. Chamberlain is the first of English statesmen to ally himself actively with our profession,
the first with imagination enough to apprehend the
great part which medical science is playing in the
world already, and to realise that only by medicine
can vast surfaces of the earth be made habitable by
white men, and those " great assets of civilisation,"
the officers of our colonies, be saved alive.   It seems
to me then that the present is a critical moment in
the relations of medicine and surgery, especially in
England where the two branches of the art have
been so radically separated as to be regarded as
" two professions "; a moment when it is our duty
to contemplate the unity of Medicine, to forecast its
development as a connected whole, and to conceive

ST. PHILIP'S COLLEGE LIBRARY

a rational ideal of its means and ends.   But this large and prophetic vision of Medicine we cannot attain without a thoughtful study of its past.

If thus, as from a height, we contemplate the story of the world, not its pageants, for in their splendour our eyes are dimmed, but the gathering, propagation and ordination of its forces, whence they sprang, and how they blend this way and that to build the institutions of men, we wonder at their creative energy, or weep over the errors and the failures, the spoliation and the decay, which have marred or thwarted them ; and if we contemplate not the whole but some part of men's sowing and men's harvest, such as Medicine, the intenser is our sorrow and disappointment, or our joy and hope, as we admire the great ends we have gained, or dwell upon the loss and suffering which have darkened the way.   In the development of Medicine, said Helmholtz, "there lies a great lesson on the true principles of scientific progress." [1]

Pray do not fear however lest, to fulfil the meaning of the title of this address, I should describe to you the history of medicine, and the history of surgery, and on this double line compare and combine my researches ; in the time allotted to me no such survey is possible.   I can but select certain eminent features of the histories of these departments of knowledge, and compare them with a view to edification; your fear may be rather lest I should

[1] ("Es liegt eine grosse Lehre über die wahren Prinzipien wissenschaftlicher Forschung in dem Entwickelungsgange der Medizin.")

ST. PHILIP'S COLLEGE LIBRARY

dress an arbitrary story with the unrighteousness of a man with a moral.

In his address on Morgagni, at Rome in 1894, Virchow said that Medicine is remarkable in its unbroken development for twenty-five centuries; as we may say without irreverence, from Hippocrates to Virchow himself. However the great pathologist's opinion seems to need severe qualification; if so it be, the stream has more than once flowed long underground. The discontinuity of Medicine from Egypt to Crotona and Ionia is even greater than from Galen to Avicenna, a period during which, in spite of a few eminent physicians in the Byzantine Empire, it sank into a sterile and superstitious routine.

Classical medicine, the medicine of the fifth century B.C., is represented for us by the great monument of the scriptures collected under the name of the foremost teacher of his age, Hippocrates; in genius perhaps the greatest physician of all past time. The treatises of the Canon may be divided into medicine, surgery, and obstetrics. The medical treatises, when read in an historical spirit, command our reverent admiration. Written at a time when an inductive physiology was out of reach, we are impressed nevertheless by their broad, rational, and almost scientific spirit. Medicine, even when not dominated by contemporary philosophy, has always taken its colour from it; and the working physiology of Hippocrates was that humoral doctrine, originally derived from

Egypt and the East, which, as enlarged by Galen, ruled over medicine ·till recent times. That in later ages it became the engine of a fantastic and tyrannous dogmatism we know but too well; how was it then that Hippocrates and his school were so little perverted by it ? To pretend that it had no such effect, or that the speculative schools of Greece swept over medicine without perverting it, would be idle. Hippocrates, while distinguishing between the methods of outward and inward maladies (φανερὰ καὶ ἄδηλα νοσήματα), taught that even for the inner many facts are accessible to methodical investigation, by careful sight and touch, laborious inspection of excretions and so forth ; yet as in these diseases the field of inference is much larger than in the outward, the data even of direct observation fell the more readily into the scheme of the four humours, and by this doctrine were so coloured that, although noted and pondered with rare clinical insight, they were read into the scheme of a fictitious pathology.

How was it then, I repeat, that the speculative side of the medicine of the period bewildered Hippocrates so little ? Because in the first instance the clinical method of the school was broadly and soundly based upon the outward maladies. No sooner did an internal affection—empyema for example—work outwards than the mastery of Hippocrates became manifest. What we moderns separate as surgery, surgery which from Galen to Paré, by Clerks, Faculties and Humanists, was despised as vile, and from Paré to Hunter as

illiberal, was in the age of Hippocrates, as in all
epochs of medicine since that age, its saviour.   By
his surgery it was that Hippocrates was led to
announce clearly and categorically the first principles
of inductive research and practice; namely, phenomena first, then judgment, then general propositions,
then practical knowledge and craft.   One principle
only, but that a great one, was wanting to him,
namely, experimental verification ; a principle not
definitely apprehended by Aristotle, nor by any
ancient physician except Galen.

If our admiration of the inner medicine of
Hippocrates, great as it is, is a relative admiration,
an admiration of the historical sense, of his outer
medicine our admiration is immediate and unqualified.   Little as the fifth century knew of
inward anatomy, as compared with Alexandria
about two centuries later, yet the marvellous eye
and touch of the Greek physician had made an
anatomy of palpable parts—a clinical anatomy—
sufficient to establish a Medicine of such parts of
the body of which our own generation would not
be ashamed.   That this acuteness of the " cerebral "
as well as of the " retinal eye," was a note of the
time, is illustrated by the observation, by Professor
Waldstein, in sculpture of this period, of a certain
muscle of the groin, especially developed no doubt
by Greek athletics, which in its now diminished
form had escaped the eyes of modern anatomists.

In respect of fractures and luxations of the
forearm M. Pétrequin pronounces Hippocrates more
complete than Boyer; in respect of congenital

luxations richer than Dupuytren. Malgaigne again
admires his comparison of the effects of unreduced
luxations on the bones, muscles, and functions of
the limb, in adults, in young children, and before
birth, as a wonderful piece of clinics.   In Littré's
judgment the work of Hippocrates on the joints is
a work for all time.   In gibbous spine he dis-
tinguishes the traumatic kind from that of internal
origin; and points out that in this case tubercles
are often found in the lungs and mediastinum, and
may indeed by extension be the direct cause of the
spinal affection; a doctrine accepted by Galen, and
then forgotten till it was recalled by Zachary Platner
early in the eighteenth century, and re-established
by Delpech in the second half of the nineteenth.
Hippocrates chides those blunderers who take a
spinal apophysis for the body of the vertebra, or
the internal tubercle of the humerus for a part of
the forearm.   On wounds, which in warlike and
unruly ages have constituted a principal branch
of surgery, Littré pronounces that the Hippocratic
books must be studied with deep attention; for
they are founded on a wide experience, minute and
profound observation, and an enlightened and infinitely cautious judgment.   In the handling of
wounds the surgeons of the Hippocratic school
were indeed, as we shall see presently, far better
instructed than the surgeons of the medieval and
renaissance periods.   If poultices were used they
were applied near but not upon the wound;
the water for washing the wounds, unless very
pure, was filtered and boiled; their linen dress-

ings were of new material, and the hands and nails of the operator were cleansed. Of the access of air to the wound the Greeks were very jealous, a jealousy which in later times led to abuse of the suture. Their local medications were wine and oil, with some excess in oil; greasy applications, or salves, became the curse of later surgery. In fresh wounds healing by first intention was expected, though in less recent and in contused wounds suppuration was anticipated. To foul wounds certain balsams were applied. Wound-fever was known to the school, and the different significance of fever in the first week and in later weeks was pointed out. Puerperal fever was interpreted as a wound-fever, and its occasional origin in retention of putrid uterine contents was recognised. In wounds of the head Hippocrates warns against careless interference with the temporal regions, lest convulsions and palsy occur on the opposite side of the body; for the trepan was then in vogue, as it had been from the darkest backward of time. In spinal injury he notes that incontinence of urine and faeces is of fatal augury. From amputation of the larger limbs he flinched, as did most if not all responsible surgeons down to Paré; for inner anatomy was ill-known, and ligature of arteries, even in wounds, made slow way : indeed before Celsus this method seems to have been unknown. Caries was not definitely distinguished from necrosis ; but a case of disease of the palate with fallen nose irresistibly suggests syphilis. On eye diseases we find much of interest, though the

media were imperfectly distinguished, and the seat
of cataract was undetected. Nyctalopia however
was recognised; and relief was given by operation
for such diseases as ectropion, hypopyon, and the
like. Of obstetrical practice, I must be content to
say that it had reached a high standard; when
surgery flourishes obstetrics flourish. By the very
wealth of knowledge in these treatises indeed we
realise that the Father of Medicine stood in the
line of a noble ancestry; and that by his genius
and leadership what I may call a great Paradosis
received a permanent form.

It is by comparison of one part of the Hippocratic Canon with another that we learn how a
strong grasp of inner medicine was attained by way
of severe discipline on its positive or surgical side.
And this not by mere empiricism; it may well have
been from Hippocrates himself that Aristotle learned
how by empiricism ($\dot{\epsilon}\mu\pi\epsilon\iota\rho\dot{\iota}a$) we perceive a certain
remedy to be good for this person or for that—for
Socrates, let us say, or for Callias—when he has
a certain fever; but by reason we discover the
characteristic common to these particular persons
whereby they react alike. In his Book of Precepts
Hippocrates tells us that $\tau\rho\iota\beta\dot{\eta}$ $\mu\epsilon\tau\dot{a}$ $\lambda\dot{o}\gamma o\nu$ is the
basis of all medical knowledge. Now $\tau\rho\iota\beta\dot{\eta}$ is
primarily a grinding or rubbing; so the student
must rub and grind at nature, using his reason at
the same time: but his reason must be a perceptive
and interpretative, not a productive faculty; for he
who lends himself to plausible ratiocination ($\lambda o\gamma\iota\sigma\mu\hat{\omega}$
$\pi\iota\theta a\nu\hat{\omega}$ $\pi\rho o\sigma\dot{\epsilon}\chi\omega\nu$) will find himself ere long in a

blind alley ; and those who have pursued this course
have done no credit to Medicine.   How soundly, for
the time, this lesson was learned we see in the
theoretical appreciation of these several faculties in
the first chapter of the *Metaphysics*, and in the
Sixth Book of the *Ethics*, where the senses, it is
urged, cannot really be separated from the mind ;
for, as St. Thomas forcibly reiterated, the senses
and the mind contribute each an element to every
knowledge.[1]   I would venture to suggest that this
method of observation, experience, and judgment
was established in Medicine first, because Medicine
of all arts is the most practical and imperative ;
and, as Aristotle says, is concerned with the individual patient : thus to our art may belong the
honour of the first application of positive methods
to all subjects of natural knowledge.

The chief lesson of the Hippocratic period for
us is that, in practice as in honour, medicine and
surgery were then one.   The Greek physician had
no more scruple in using his hands in the service
of his brains than had Pheidias or Archimedes ;
and it was by this co-operation that in the fifth
century an advance was achieved which in our
eyes is marvellous.   As we pursue the history of
medicine in later times we shall see the error, the
blindness, and even the degradation of the physicians
who neglected and despised a great handicraft.   To
the clear eyes of the ancient Greeks an art was
not liberal or illiberal by its manipulations but by
its ends.   As because of its ends the cleansing and

---

[1] Compare also the last chapter of the *Posterior Analytics*.

solace of the lepers by St. Basil, St. Francis and
Father Damien was a service of angels, so Hippocrates saw no baseness even in manipulations which
obtained for his followers the name of *coprophagi* :
where there is no overcoming there is no victory.

Between Hippocrates and Galen, an interval of
some five centuries, flourished the great anatomical and
medical schools of Alexandria. Our only important
source however for the medicine of the Alexandrian
period is Celsus, who lived in the reign of Augustus.
From Celsus we infer indeed that the brilliant
anatomy of Alexandria made for good practice in
surgery, and for surgical diagnosis; yet the influence seems not to have been so direct and effective
as might be supposed.   Haeser argues indeed that
too intense a devotion to healing as a craft prevented the healer from thinking anatomically.   As
regards the Empirical School this may be true ; for
by it not only was systematic thinking discouraged,
but ancillary science was regarded also as vain, if
not mischievous.   Its spokesman Serapion protested,
against the great anatomists, that in Medicine
observation and record are all-sufficient.   This was
to look at nature indeed, but with the many faceted
eye of the insect.   No doubt with the exception of
anatomy the ancillary sciences were in a vaporous
condition, and to the hardihood of the empirics,
narrow as it was, medicine owed much.   Still, as
facts will return in ever new combinations they
must provisionally be interpreted by analogy ; that
is, by the application of universals from one sphere

to another. Thus in *Airs, Waters, and Places* analogy was safer for Hippocrates than a rudimentary geography and meteorology, and, as is notable in his school, it did good service in prognosis ; yet analogy is so facile an instrument that even in the school of Hippocrates the temptation to use it became too strong and too general. Inductive in spirit analogy may be, as even Serapion (in his " ἡ τοῦ ὁμοίου μετάβασις ") admitted ; but it lends itself very freely to airy and even to metaphysical hypotheses, wares which can be turned out in satisfactory profusion without that πεῖρα τριβική—that grinding and rubbing in nature—on which Hippocrates insisted. For the solid work of surgery and midwifery, however, such fabrics are too flimsy ; they find their market in inner medicine, a domain in which, as surgeons in all times have been wont to complain, our failures are covered up and buried.

Nevertheless in the VIIth and VIIIth Books of Celsus we see that surgery and midwifery had made substantial progress since Hippocrates, and probably since the Alexandrine School of Erasistratus and Herophilus. Celsus, probably not himself a practitioner,[1] is rather vague in detail : still,

[1] In deference to the opinion of the last editors of Celsus, Angiolo and Isidoro Del Lungo, who opine that Celsus was himself formally a practitioner of Medicine, I changed the "probably not" of my manuscript into "perhaps not." But on further consideration of the arguments of the Del Lungos I have returned to "probably not." What Scaliger and Casaubon thought may on this point have little weight with us ; that Morgagni regarded Celsus as a practising physician has no doubt far more. Still Daremberg [the standard Latin text is that of Daremberg (Leipzig, 1859)], Pidoux, Broca, Védrènes, have decided otherwise ; and although I cannot set my superficial impressions of this author beside the ripe studies of Angiolo Del Lungo, yet I cannot help coming also to

besides the Hippocratic surgery, we recognise means
of treatment in piles, fistula, rodent ulcer, eczema,
fractures, and luxations ; missiles were removed
from their wounds ; tumours—of which surgeons
before and after were afraid—were excised ; the
nasal passages were cauterised for ozæna ; dropsies
were systematically tapped ; hernias were submitted
to radical cure ; genito-urinary diseases were attacked
in both sexes ; his operation for stone, as we shall
see, held the field till Malgaigne and Cheselden ;
plastic operations were undertaken ; arteries were
tied, and, for the first time, the larger limbs were
deliberately amputated—though only in extreme
need, and often with fatal results by secondary
hæmorrhage and otherwise. His wound surgery was
Hippocratic (p. 8), and he warns the surgeon, in his
anxiety to exclude the air, not to use the suture
until the depth of the wound has been so cleansed
that no clot remains, for this turns into pus, excites
inflammation and prevents union. These chapters
signify a large accumulation of experience on a
positive method, which can hardly be predicated of
the inner medicine of the period.[1]

the opinion that in some places Celsus speaks as a physician would
hardly have spoken, and in other and not a few places omits, to
one's vexation, those intimate details which a practical man would
surely have made a point of. And how strange it is that no one
of the physicians of the later Empire—Greek physicians, it is true,
but again that neither Pliny nor Quintilian—alludes to Celsus as a
practitioner ; strangely inconsistent as this calling would have been
with the prejudices of his class in Rome. Furthermore, we know that
Celsus wrote "non sine cultu et nitore" (Quintilian) like treatises on
agriculture, rhetoric, law, philosophy, and the art of war. Celsus,
it would seem, preceded Robert Pullen and Brunetto Latini as an
encyclopedist. After all the matter is not worth much ink.

[1] Recent excavations have yielded a rich collection of surgical

How active surgery was from Celsus to Galen, and how honourable and progressive a part of Medicine, we know from the scanty records handed down to us in the compilations of Oribasius and other authors. From the remnants of the writings of Heliodorus we gather many things; among others that amputation was resorted to in comminuted fracture — *e.g.* of the leg below the knee — before gangrene actually set in; moreover that the operation was very carefully performed, including the preparation of some sort of flaps. Archigenes of Apamea also practised in Rome, in the reign of Trajan. Galen calls him an acute but too subtle a physician; such of his subtilties as are known to us however — his distinction between primary and consequential symptoms for instance — are to his credit. He applied the ligature in amputations; and that remarkable man Antyllus, who unfortunately is known to us only in Oribasius and his copyist Paul,[1] applied the method to the cure of aneurysm, which however Rufus seems to have done before him. Galen tells us where he got his " Celtic linen thread " for the purpose, namely " at a shop in the Via Sacra between the Temple of Rome and the Forum ": a shop near his own house, which was

instruments which are a vivid illustration of the ingenious and methodical surgery of the Roman Empire. In his edition of Celsus M. Védrènes publishes plates of these, and uses them aptly in the interpretation of the author.

[1] That Paul in the seventh century may have had direct access to extant works of Antyllus is possible; but the manner of his citation is that of a copyist, and in matter coincides with the selections of Oribasius. I ought to say that Haeser gives Paul more credit for originality than I am yet able to do.

also in the Via Sacra, by the Temple of Peace.
We learn also, from Oribasius, that Antyllus practised extensive resections of bone in the limbs,
and even in the upper and lower jaw.   Much excellent surgery, of which I cannot now speak in
detail, disappeared in the chaos of the Dark Ages.

Galen came to Rome under Marcus Aurelius.
In the biological sciences this great physician
stands to Harvey as in physics Archimedes stood
to another great physician, William Gilbert; Galen
was the first, as for many centuries he was the last,
to apply the experimental method to physiology.
He embraced the ancillary sciences; he opened
out new routes and he improved the old.   Unhappily his soaring genius took delight also in
the spheres of speculation; and it was not the
breadth of his science nor the depth of his
methodical experiment, but the height of his
visionary conceits which imposed upon the Middle
Ages.   Galen did not himself forget the precept
of Hippocrates—To look, to touch, to hear (" καὶ
ἰδεῖν, καὶ θιγεῖν, καὶ ἀκοῦσαι"); but he did not
wholly subdue himself to the πεῖρα τριβική—
this toilsome conversation with troublesome facts.
For example; in a pseudo-galenist treatise, but
one which fairly represents what we know of
Galen's doctrines,[1] we read . . . " προηγεῖται δὲ τῆς
πράξεως ἡ θεωρία . . . ἀρχὴ γὰρ τῆς ἐπὶ τῶν
ἔργων τριβῆς ἡ διὰ τοῦ λόγου διδασκαλία."   Nay,
possessed by platonist visions, enamoured of an

---

[1] *Definitiones medicae*, Ed. Kühn, xix. 351. Palissy said his
proofs were "*la veue, l'ouye et l'attouchement.*"

elaborate teleology of his own, and in violent reaction against the Empirics, he formulated an
eclectic doctrine contrary to the experimental reason
(τριβὴ μετὰ λόγου); and taught categorically that
speculation shall guide experience.   So it was that
he imposed philosophical lectures upon students as
preliminary to medical study, carried speculation
into his physiological experiments and even into
anatomy itself, gave a subjective cast to his finest
work, and foisted metaphysics in another guise on
medicine.   Galen did not make any great mark on
surgery.   He followed Hippocrates in the distinction
between healing by first and second intention, and,
to promote healing by first intention, in desiring a
clean and dry wound, with good apposition for exclusion of air.   His tracts on the eye are lost; but,
so far as we know, his surgery was adopted in the
main from the Alexandrians, and from Soranus.
However, Galen successfully resected the sternum
for caries, exposing the heart ; and he excised a
splintered shoulder blade : moreover, with all his
bent to speculative reason, we have no hint that he
fell into the medieval abyss of regarding surgery as
unfit for a scholar and a gentleman.

As a positive discipline the diseases of women
may be counted with surgery; but within our limits
that subject cannot be discussed separately.   However it would never do to omit the name of no less
a physician of the time—Soranus of Ephesus—
who, by the accident of surviving records, is
chiefly associated with these diseases.   Soranus
practised at Rome under Trajan and Hadrian, and

was therefore a contemporary of Archigenes, and little older than Galen. If in breadth of thought and swiftness of invention Soranus pales before Galen, yet in sober moments we may be tempted to regard him as the greater physician. In any case he must rank with Galen as one of the greatest physicians of antiquity. If the Methodists, of whom Soranus was the chief, fashioned for themselves the yoke of " strictum and laxum " as the poles of a new physiology, yet it is not easy to say that by this doctrine they were more entangled than were the dogmatists by the humoral doctrine, than was Hoffmann by " tone and atony," or the other systematists of the eighteenth century by their respective notions; physicians, many of them at any rate, masters in medicine nevertheless. The treatise of Soranus on Diseases of Women may be ranked with the surgical treatises of Hippocrates as a classic which no lapse of time can efface ; and if on the degree of his influence as a general surgeon, and on those remnants of his surgical writings which have floated down to us on such rafts as Aetius and Paul of Egina, we have to assign to Soranus a place much lower than Hippocrates, yet his place was considerable enough to testify that in the Empire, as in Ionia and Alexandria, Medicine was saved by the honour and vitality of its surgery from the fictions and the petrifactions of philo-sophical systems. If in many directions, as for instance in the treatment of empyema, Soranus evidently fell behind Hippocrates, on the detail of

operations for hernia, and even for stone, he was
clearer than Celsus.

After Galen and Soranus Medicine came to
the evening of its second day, to the long night
before the rise of the Arabian, Italian, and French
surgeons of the thirteenth and fourteenth centuries.
By the divulsion of the Empire, by the degradation
of morals to which even Pliny and Galen had begun
to bear witness, and by the inroads of barbarians,
arts and sciences were trampled under foot in the
West until by the iron scaffold of the Faith a new
society should be erected.   In the East was more
tranquillity; and the night was illumined by
moons, such as Oribasius, Alexander of Tralles,
and Paul of Egina, by whose reflected light men
groped their way.   To these physicians our debt
is rather one of preservation of good tradition than
of discovery.   Alexander was no great surgeon; but
he tells us of the diagnosis of ascites by percussion,
of anasarca by pitting, of large spleen by palpation;
and he makes some shrewd remarks on urinary sedi-
ments: still all these were parts no doubt of the
current knowledge of his time.   Such swallows
made no summer; and their work lies out of my
argument that surgery, though scorned by the high
stomachs of the Middle Ages, has never been the
child or the humble companion of medicine but
the stone of the corner and the key to its true
method.

Not only did Greek Medicine reach the medieval
physicians in a fragmentary, mutilated and per-

verted form, but in this form Medicine came to them untempered. A mutilated and special tradition was separated from the organism of Greek accomplishment ; it was deprived of the Greek breadth of thought, of the Greek spirit of intellectual freedom. Remnants of Greek lore, thus distorted never coherent, lay heavily upon minds unprepared to assimilate or use them. The mystical tendency of thought in the Middle Ages, the disposition to ontological absoluteness, the reliance upon precision of argument as the means of attaining truth, the transfusion of doctrine with Eastern fantasies, made of the Greek Medicine a widely different and far less scientific conception. By its ontological form medieval thought led to the idea of a wound as an entity having a substantial existence apart from or imposed upon the body ; and, as such, possessed of its own modes and phases of life, modes and phases susceptible of independent fashion and direction under the hand of the physician. Moreover the scholastic tendency to dialectical subtilties led to an elaboration of factitious schedules and nomenclatures of these modes and phases, which enthralled the faculty of observation ; while the mysticism manifested itself in magic, in egregious medicines and in barbarous perplexities of ingredients.

Thus it came about that in spite of the docile industry of certain physicians of the Byzantine period, medicine gradually sank not into sterility only but into deep degradation : for the wholesome discipline of practical surgery had fallen off. Eastern folk, who bear heaven - sent sores with fatal stoicism, repel

the profane hand of man;[1] and the tradition of
Galen made for a plague of drugs which were least
mischievous when merely superfluous. Nor was an
overloaded and a filthy pharmacy the only sorrow
of the sick; as art grew empty, sorcery, demonology
and astrology entered more and more into the void.
The Saracens, keen and intelligent as they were,
and rich as were their gifts to the West, did little
to remove and something perhaps to favour the
aversion from surgery, and the social contempt of it,
which culminated in the ban of the Council of Tours.
Under the sanctions of Islam anatomy was impossible. By the door of the East, Rhazes, Albucasis,
Avicenna—the Arabian Galen, had entered into
a great scientific inheritance; and though they
did not do much, it is true, to ennoble surgery,
yet with them it was a grave and an honourable
calling; with them Medicine had not yet lopped off
her right arm. The Danaan gifts of the Western
Church to Medicine issued in a far worse treachery.
The Greek of Ireland, and of England in the time
of Bede, was banished by Augustine and the Bene-
dictine missionaries; and the medicine of Monte
Cassino, itself indeed but a farrago of receipts, fell
lower and lower in the monkish hostels of the
West.[2] We have reason however to believe that

[1] In modern Islam I understand Medicine is now almost wholly
in the hands of the barbers; the actual cautery is in much
request; and cutting for stone, and operation for cataract are in
the hands of specialists as they were from time immemorial in the
West. Some of these customs are evident, even to the passing
traveller, in Algeria, Tunisia, or Egypt.

[2] Before printing medical precepts were often put into verse, an
aid to memory which it is not for us to scoff at; though when in

some fair surgery persisted, even in the cloister, until it was formally abandoned to the "secular arm" in A.D. 1163;[1] and books on surgery and midwifery began to disappear from conventual libraries. About the same time the University of Paris excluded all those who worked with their hands;[2] so that students of medicine had to abjure manual occupation, and to content themselves with syllogisms and inspections of urine, often without any inspection of the patient himself. From the University the Faculty of Medicine took its tone, and the surgical corporation of St. Côme aped the Faculty (p. 59). But by the expulsion of surgery from the liberal arts Medicine herself was eviscerated; the pernicious bisection of Medicine was made

the third century one Serenus Samonicus wrote *De medicina praecepta saluberrima*, in 1115 clumsy hexameters, we can scarcely wonder that Caracalla had him destroyed. Early in the twelfth century Odo de Meudon, or de Meune, wrote in poetry on 65 herbs and 12 medicines (Haeser); and the medical poetry of Gilles de Corbeuil, body physician of Philip Augustus, "De urinis" and "De pulsibus," and the versifications of Salerno are well known. (Cf. Kühn, *Abh. z. Gesch. d. Med.* Heft viii. 1904). Unfortunately even Fracastoro chose this fanciful shape for his work on Syphilis, and was hymned in English by Nahum Tate.

[1] The Rheims (A.D. 1125) and Lateran (A.D. 1139) Councils restricted the surgery of the clerical or, in other words, of the educated class, and no doubt feudal ideas did no less to abase its services; it was at Tours however that the sinister and perfidious "ecclesia abhorret a sanguine" was first pronounced.

[2] The denunciations of the Faculty of Medicine in Paris were almost as appalling as those of Ernulphus: *e.g.* "Famosum libellum mendacibus conviciis, impudentibus calumnis refertum," etc. etc. "Ipsum Torquetum indignum judicat, qui nequam medicinam faciat, propter temeritatem, impudentiam et verae medicinae ignorantiam . . . ipsum Torquetum similiaque hominum et opinionum portenta a se suisque finibus arceant," etc. etc. This specimen is of the late fifteenth century but is no unfair instance of the spirit of the University of Paris in the Middle Ages.

which has not yet spent its evil : the very foundation of the art was gone, and the clergy and the
faculties, in France and England at any rate,
devoted all their energies to shoring up the
superstructure.   Surgery had its revenge, its bitter
revenge ; but in the desecration of its own temple.

In the thirteenth and fourteenth centuries
however surgery, hated and avoided by Medical
Faculties, scorned in clerical and feudal circles,
began in the hands of lowly and unlettered men
to grow from the root ; while inward medicine,
withdrawing itself more and more from the sources
and the laboratory of nature, hardened into the
shell which till the seventeenth century bore but a
false counterfeit of life.   The surgeons of the
thirteenth, fourteenth and fifteenth centuries,
reared in base apprenticeships, not only illiterate
but forbidden even the means of learning, lay
under heavy disadvantages ; yet by practical experience and technical resource they were making
the future of our art.   Towards the end of the
fifteenth century indeed even this progress had
slackened ; it was soon reinforced however by
new and urgent problems, not of the schools
but of direct rough and tumble with nature : of
these new problems, of which Paré became the
chief interpreter, the wounds of firearms were
perhaps the most urgent.

It is remarkable that around the papal chair
the velvet of the hand of the Church was
thicker than the iron.   In the air of Rome or of
Avignon the grim rigour of Paris was marvellously

softened.   In Bologna, Padua and Montpellier
Medicine could develop, if not freely, yet in
tranquillity, and undivided.   The peace of Con-
stance (A.D. 1183) had enfranchised the great
Italian cities, and a truce with the Empire gave
to lay and clerical potentates time and occasion for
the foundation of universities.   In Italy the unity
of Medicine, as in Greek and Latin ages, was still
preserved : in Bologna there were indeed physicians
and surgeons and barbers, but divisions had not
yet gone deep ; the titles melted into one another.
In the twelfth century Gerard of Cremona, the
translator of the Arabian versions of Greek
Medicine, who by the frank and discreet selection
of his authors did more for North Italy than
Constantine had done in the eleventh for Monte
Cassino and South Italy, rendered the surgical
treatise of Albucasis (p. 44) into latin ; and he left
his books to the convent of St. Lucia, where he
was buried : now in those days to a school books
were a fortune.[1]   With the rise of Bologna, and
the richer endowments of its chairs, the school
of Salerno, the oldest medical school of modern
Europe, but the poorest in the books of the best
Arab physicians, began to diminish ; and Bologna,
quickly surpassing the other Italian schools,
now rivalled Montpellier and Paris.   In Medicine
indeed Italy[2] then led the world ; in the great
schools of Salerno, Naples, Bologna, Padua, there

[1] In the thirteenth century a learned Spanish Jew, Ferraguth,
made the most important contributions from the Arabian schools.

[2] Italy had at this period a far wider and keener sense of unity
than in later centuries.

was contained a strong lay and imperial tradition, which arrested hieratic ascendancy. Moreover latin medical prose, which was not established in France, England, or Germany till the middle of the thirteenth century,[1] was forming in Italy, even in the eleventh, upon the latin renderings of Arab versions of the Greek physicians; a condition of progress as vital for the time as the rise of the vernaculars in the fourteenth (p. 81).

Before the rise of Padua, Bologna was indeed a large and plenteous mother to Medicine in her full orb; yet even in Salerno far-seeing men had begun to dread the divorce of surgery from medicine. In the middle of the thirteenth century Bruno, a Calabrian probably educated at Salerno, in his "*Chirurgia Magna*," a work which, although a motley blend of Hippocrates, Galen, Paul of Egina and the Arabs, was that of a learned and experienced man, bitterly resents the separation of medicine from surgery by celibate clerks who in false squeamishness shirked operations.[2]   Even

[1] This great service was of course first undertaken by Celsus, and performed consummately; though where latin fell short he had to insert "quod Graeci vocant" and the like. But, as the eminent physicians of the Empire after his time were Greeks, Celsus, to the grievous misfortune of Europe, was practically forgotten till Thomas of Sarzanne's (afterwards Nicholas V.) discovery of the Ambrosian manuscript (p. 55) in 1443. Nevertheless from some hints of Cassiodorus, which are possibly allusions to Celsus, and again of Gerbert (Sylvester II.) it would seem that even in the tenth century Celsus was read in some monastic libraries. On the other hand his treatise was printed as early as 1478 and sixty latin editions followed between that date and the time of Fabricius who declared:—"Admirabilis Celsus in omnibus, quem nocturna versare manu, versare diurno consulo." How Morgagni studied Celsus, and enriched his work with commentaries, is still better known. Aretæus was little known in the Middle Ages.

[2] Yet even in early Salernitan times there was a class of inferior

in Italy the clergy carried much weight in university graduation, and the students in all faculties bore the tonsure. And if Papal Bulls conferred privileges, they usually implied or imposed restrictions. When in some places a lower examination was provided for unclerkly, that is in other words, illiterate, persons desiring to practise as surgeons only, the wedge was driven in deeper. The important Salernitan treatise—*The Glosses of the Four Masters on the Surgery of Roger and Roland*, edited by Daremberg and de Renzi, begins with regretting the decadence of surgery, which these masters attribute to two causes ; namely, the division of surgery from medicine, and the neglect of anatomy. By the wisdom of Bologna and Naples, where were founded chairs of surgery, this ill-starred divorce was postponed ; in his University of Naples indeed Frederick the Second made it a condition that surgery should be an essential part of Medicine, should occupy as long a course of study, and should be founded on anatomy " without which no operator can be successful."

The School of Salerno was the first renascence of clinical experience ; and Roger, the Salernitan, and Roland of Parma, upon whose surgery was founded the commentary of The Four Masters,[1]

barbers or surgeons ; for Bruno himself, while claiming the right of performing "all operations," yet in respect of minor practice excuses himself thus : "praeterquam de scarificatione et flebotomia, que licet cyrurgie species habeantur . . . noluerunt medici propter indecentiam exercere sed illas barberiorum in manibus reliquerunt." (Quoted by Julius Pagel in Puschmann's *Handbuch*.)

[1] In Cambridge we have two MSS. of the Four Masters ; that in the Peterhouse Library being the finer example. It is a folio

stand like Twin Brethren in the dawn of modern
Medicine, bearing the very names of romance.
Roger's "*Practica Chirurgiae*" was written in 1180,
and was re-edited by Roland nearly a hundred years
later. It was no mere recooking of Albucasis:
although of course it rests upon the traditional
surgery of his day, there are not a few points of
interest in the book, such as certain descriptions
suggestive of syphilis. Under the title of the
paragraph — for it is no more — *De cancro in
virga virili,* carcinoma is included, but probably
syphilis also. In some of these cases they tell us
phagedena ensued. Before Theodoric, Roger refrac-
tured badly united bones. For hæmorrhage he
used styptics, the suture, or the ligature; the
ligature he learned no doubt from Paul: but
Roger, like most or all qualified practitioners
of the period, was a "wound-surgeon"; that is
he did not undertake the larger operations. He
warns against operating in cancer, especially if of

on vellum, written in a good fourteenth century hand, and evidently
not a scholar's but a professor's copy. It is neatly illuminated
and rubricated. The title is *Cirurgia iiii magistrorum cum
additionibus Rolandi.* The volume contains in the first place
the "Breviarius Constantini qui dicitur viaticus, cum glossulis
Gerardi." This work extends to 143 ff., that of the Four Masters
to about 30. One may see that Roger's tract on surgery owes much
to Constantine's *Viaticum.* Who the four masters were who
developed Roger's tract into a still more interesting work is mere
speculation. Roland's additions were composed in 1264. The
Peterhouse scribe entitles the work as of Mag. Rogerus and three
others, and gives 1230 A.D. as the date of its appearance. This
may have been the date of the early (original ?) copy now in
Florence (Libr. Magliabecchi). This I have not seen, but I understand that this copy Mag. Guido aretinus (Arensium) "correxit et
manifestavit," and it is to the care of this editor that the Peterhouse text is attributed.

uterus or rectum.   He was in favour, as a rule, of
immediate extraction of weapons from their wounds;
in these wounds, even after extrusion of the foreign
body, he promoted coction or suppuration, and
dressed them with galenical salves on lint.   His
bandaging seems to have been very efficient.   To
these points especially—to the withdrawal of the
weapon, to the promotion of pus, and to unctuous
dressings—I would call your attention; for now
we are approaching more nearly the controversy
which, pale reflexion as it may be of the great
surgical regeneration of the nineteenth century, is,
historically speaking, of singular interest.   Less
blessed than we, our fathers determined this controversy the wrong way, and thereby brought upon
themselves, and upon their children for many
generations, malpractices and tortures which—or
so it seems to us—a contrary decision would have
averted.

Let us now return to Bologna.   Hugh of
Lucca, says Malgaigne, is the first of the surgeons
of modern Europe whom we can cite with honour.
This tribute is a little strained; we may say,
however, that of these honourable ancestors Hugh
seems to have been the greatest.   I say "seems to
have been"; for Hugh is even a dimmer giant
than Roger or Roland.   We know that he served
as surgeon in campaigns, and was present at the
siege of Damietta; but of writing he left not a
line.   Such vision as we have of him we owe to
his loyal disciple, perhaps his son, the Dominican
Theodoric (Teodorico Borgognoni: A.D. 1205-1296),

Bishop of Cervia near Ravenna, confessor of Innocent IV.,[1] and the master of Henry of Mondeville. From Lucca Theodoric extended his practice far and wide, and, as Haeser remarks, made the noblest use of his earnings. He completed his treatise in 1266.[2] Salernitan practice needed the reforms of Theodoric " qui pulcherrimas cicatrices sine unguento aliquo inducebat." After some reference to Theodoric's work and a close study of Henry of Mondeville and Guy of Chauliac, I am of Haeser's opinion that Guy dealt with Theodoric unfairly; and, I would add, not only unfairly but even disastrously. What the later history of surgery might have been had that illustrious surgeon been more illustrious still, and carried forward the reform of Hugh, Theodoric, and Henry, is one of those historical speculations which may be left to the curious; the history of what has not happened cannot occupy much of the attention of serious students. It is sufficient to say that the judicious Guy held to galenism and to coction or suppuration, and rivetted upon surgery the grievous orthodoxy of which it had not purged itself even in the days of the studentship of many of us now living.[3]

What was Theodoric's message ? He wrote :—

[1] I give the current story, but there is some evidence of two Theodorics—the Bishop, and a surgeon, by birth a Catalan.

[2] Dr. Payne (FitzPatrick Lectures for 1904) says that Theodoric took his description of leprosy from Gilbertus Anglicus, a description evidently at first hand, and in many respects very accurate.

[3] Dr. Ernst Becker in his interesting tract on Medicine in medieval Hildesheim (Berlin, 1899) in estimating the value of medical fees in the fifteenth century says we must remember the long duration of attendances "bei der wohl regelmässig eintretenden Eiterung aller Wunden."

" for it is not necessary, as Roger and Roland have written, as many of their disciples teach, and as all modern surgeons profess, that pus should be generated in wounds. No error can be greater than this. Such a practice is indeed to hinder nature, to prolong the disease, and to prevent the conglutination and consolidation of the wound." (Book II. c. 27.)   In principle what more did Lister say than this ?   Henry of Mondeville made a hard fight for the new principle, but the advocates of suppuration won all along the line ; and for centuries to come poultices and grease were still to be applied to fresh wounds ; and tents, plastered with irritants to promote suppuration, were still to be thrust into the recesses of them, even when there was no foreign matter to be discharged.   If after all this erysipelas set in— well, says Henry, we will lay it at the door of St. Eligius !

It·is not easy to trace the growth of opinion on the process of healing by suppuration.   The Hippo-cratic schools are responsible for the original form of the doctrine of the four humours and for the conception of crudity and coction ; but in this school, and probably in Alexandria, if we may judge by Celsus, the practice of wound surgery was, as I have said (p. 8), sound on the whole. Speculation was not allowed to vitiate positive and direct experience.   It must not be forgotten that suppuration was a rude method of expelling the foulness of wounds ; but we must attribute the enormous vogue of treating wounds by salves and

sophistry, to the medieval travesty of Galen, and to
that galenical machine which, in the manufacture
of opinion, was as exacting and as inveterate as
the aristotelian (p. 20). Wine was an old remedy
in wounds; before Hippocrates it was exhibited
by the Good Samaritan. Rhazes used alcohol as
an antiseptic wound-wash; but he complicated
his practice with a mystical polypharmacy. Hugh
and Theodoric denounced the suppurative remedies
and promoted healing by first intention. For the
fresh wound they rejected oils and salves as too
slippery for union, and poultices as too moist
("oleum et caetera unctuosa labefaciunt et maculant
vulnus"): they washed the wound with wine
only, scrupulously removing every foreign particle;
then they brought the edges together, forbidding
any of the wine or other dressing to remain within.
As with the genuine Hippocratic school, a dry and
adhesive edge was their desire. Nature, they said,
produces the means of union in a viscous exudation,
or balm—as Paracelsus called it, a word which Paré
and Würtz adopted. In stale wounds they did
their best to obtain union by cleansing, desiccation,
and refreshing of the edges. Upon the outer
surface they laid lint steeped in wine. Powders
however they regarded as too desiccating, for
powders thus shut in decomposing matters (" saniem
incarcerant "); wine, after washing, purifying, and
drying the raw surfaces, evaporates. The quick,
shrewd, and rational observation and the original
genius of Theodoric I would gladly illustrate
did time permit; in passing I may say that he

was the first to notice salivation as the result of administration of mercury in " skin diseases." [1]

Of the adherents of Hugh and Theodoric was the well-known Arnold of Villanova, the prototype of Basil Valentine and Paracelsus, and the champion of spirits of wine ; a visionary indeed but a man of mark. He tells us naïvely that, like all the wound surgeons of his time, he flinched from large operations because of the " venae pulsatiles " which are so dangerous, defying even the cautery. Amputations of the larger limbs, I repeat, were rarely undertaken by any kind of surgeon ; and the radical cure of hernia, cutting for stone, and eye operations were performed, often brutally enough, by travelling surgeons of the short robe, who were usually out of reach of the avenger before the result became manifest. Franco, as we shall presently see, was the first modern surgeon to raise these operations again to the standard of Celsus.

Both for his own great merits, as an original and independent observer, and as the master of Lanfranc, William Salicet (Guglielmo Salicetti of Piacenza, in latin use G. Placentinus or de Saliceto —now Cadeo) was eminent among the great Italian physicians of the latter half of the thirteenth century. Now these great Italians were as distinguished in surgery as in medicine, and William was

---

[1] Theodoric's treatise is to be found in most of the early printed collections of surgical treatises which were published in Venice : e.g. that of 1519.   I ought perhaps to say this Address was written —and indeed delivered at St. Louis, before I had lighted on the article Gesch. d. Medizin im Mittelalter in the new volume of Puschmann's Handbuch by that admirable historian Dr. Pagel.

one of the protestants of the period against the division of surgery from inner medicine ; a division which he regarded as a separation of Medicine from intimate touch with nature. Like Lanfranc and the other great surgeons of the Italian tradition, and unlike Franco and Paré, he had the advantage of the liberal university education of Italy ; but, like Paré and Würtz, he had large practical experience in hospital and in the battlefield. He practised first at Bologna, afterwards in Verona. William fully recognised that surgery cannot be learned from books only. His *Surgery* contains many case histories, for he rightly opined that good notes of cases are the soundest foundation of good practice ; and in this opinion and method Lanfranc followed him. William discovered that dropsy may be due to a " durities renum " ; he substituted the knife for the arabist abuse of the cautery ; he investigated the causes of the failure of healing by first intention; he described the danger of wounds of the neck; he sutured divided nerves ; he forwarded the diagnosis of suppurative disease of the hip ; and he referred chancre and phagedæna to " coitus cum meretrice."

Lanfranc (Lanfranchi), like William Salicet a clerkly physician, was driven from Milan by the violence of the Visconti ; he fled to Lyons, and in 1295 to Paris, where he became a founder of French surgery, and gave a temporary renown to the surgical College of St. Côme, which had then received formal institution from St. Louis. He established clinical classes, and honourably and explicitly taught in

D

them all he knew. We learn from Mondeville, and many another source, that one cause of the poverty and defect of medieval medicine lay in the jealous secretiveness of its practitioners, a reticence which they carried even into their private consultations.[1] Seeing that even the greatest of them lifted matter literally and in bulk from others without the smallest sign of acknowledgment, this reticence is scarcely surprising. Theodoric himself had deferred to put his experience into writing till his old age, and much book-making was stopped by this jealousy; a result which the hearer will regard, as his mood may be, with thankfulness or with regret.

Lanfranc's " *Chirurgia Magna* " was a great work, written by a reverent but independent follower of Salicet. He distinguished between venous and arterial hæmorrhage, and used styptics (rabbit's fur, aloes, and white of egg was a popular styptic in elder surgery), digital compression for an hour, or in severe cases ligature. His chapter on injuries of the head is one of the classics of medieval surgery. Clerk as he was, Lanfranc nevertheless saw but the more clearly the danger of

---

[1] Even in the sixteenth century no less a man than Galileo declined to make public his secret method of grinding lenses till near his death. A veterinary surgeon, who flourished greatly in Yorkshire some hundred years ago as a marvellously successful operator, astutely evaded all prying and questioning into his secret, even when in imminent peril on a bed of sickness. He survived to carry all before him for many years longer. At length, bowed down by old age and decrepitude, he was again implored by his son to tell what he did in the secret half hour before operating. Life was ebbing at last, and the worn out old man whispered with his passing breath " I biles my tools."

separating surgery from medicine. " Good God ! "
he exclaims, " why this abandoning of operations
by physicians to lay persons, disdaining surgery, as
I perceive, because they do not know how to
operate . . . an abuse which has reached such a
point that the vulgar begin to think the same man
cannot know medicine and surgery. . . . I say
however that no man can be a good physician
who has no knowledge of operative surgery ; a
knowledge of both branches is essential." *(Chir.
Magna.)* Is it not strange that this ancient was
wiser than most of us are even yet !

In the Medicine of the Netherlands one of the
pupils of Lanfranc, a Flemish physician named
Yperman, appears to have been the greatest name
before Vesalius. In the recent edition of M. Broeckx,
no doubt an excellent text, there is no translation of
the Dutch ; not even an analysis of the contents.
Now it is not given to many of us to read Dutch ;
in the midst of other tasks one can but decipher this
passage or that, in a literal way, without however
gaining a sense of the general tone or qualities of the
author.   The father of Flemish surgery was born,
probably at Ypres, at the close of the thirteenth
century.   He completed his studies in Paris, as a
pupil of Lanfranc, with whom he kept up some
friendship after his return to Ypres, where he
settled in practice.   He became entitled to be
called " Master " in the year 1303-4.   He was
not in holy orders, but was a clerk, in the sense
of academic culture and degree ; his writings indeed

reveal a learned as well as a sagacious and skilful
surgeon. In one passage he describes what a good
surgeon ought to be, and among his requirements
are grammar, rhetoric and ethics ; moreover, says
M. Broeckx, a lofty tone animates all his work.
He displays—the same critic tells us—a genius
for surgery, and sturdily held his own, even with
Lanfranc himself. Yperman describes the ligature,
and, a few lines lower down, torsion of arteries.
In two of the manuscripts, one of which I have
examined in the library of St. John's College in
Cambridge, are not a few drawings of instruments.
The date of his death is unknown. This great
surgeon, whose name won almost a proverbial
renown, worked for good in the midst of a degraded
surgery of salves and superstitions ; but his writings,
strangely enough, were lost in oblivion for six
centuries ! Copies of them in Flemish were discovered in the year 1818. It seems certain that
he wrote the first manuscript in latin, for the use of
his son ; and that later copies were written in
Flemish, but we have no copy in his own hand-
writing. That in St. John's College is evidently a
school copy, and may be compared with the much
finer MS. of Lanfranc, a professor's copy, in the
same library. Yperman wrote also a treatise, now
very incomplete, on inner medicine, which also
indicates, says Dr. Pagel,[1] considerable originality
and self-reliance. In comparing these treatises, I
am struck, in the *Medicine*, by the little reliance
he placed on the physicians ; he does not quote

[1] Puschmann's *Handbuch*, vol. i. p. 737.

more than a dozen of them; in the *Surgery* on the
other hand he quotes from surgical authors many
times on a page. May we not thus infer the
opinion of an observer so independent and penetrating as Yperman on the comparative poverty of
the medicine of the period?

The early history of French surgery, to which
after a brief digression I return, has been diminished
by the light of Paré, which eclipsed the illustrious
men who went before him and beside him; of these
indigenous French surgeons Henry of Mondeville and
Guy of Chauliac were the chief. The *Chirurgia
Magna* of Guy may be regarded indeed as the
foundation of modern surgical doctrine in Western
Europe. In Henry of Mondeville, of Montpellier
and Paris, we still find the clerkly physician who
notwithstanding vindicated for surgery its true
place in Medicine. More clear-headed in this
respect than Guy, who claimed for surgery only a
place beside medicine and coequal with it, Henry
rightly declared, with Galen, that surgery is but a
method of treatment, and belongs to all Medicine.
Haeser seems to me to do less than justice to this
hardy and original reformer, the last champion in
his day of two causes—the solidarity of Medicine,
and union by first intention; the second of these
causes was lost for 600 years, the first is not
fully won even yet. Of his student life little is
known. It seems probable that he was educated at
Montpellier, and certainly he was a pupil of Theodoric in Italy. Henry's writings, rich in mother

wit, and only too racy of worldly wisdom, are as
entertaining as they are instructive.   For their
audacity of opinion and biting satire they were
displeasing to the Church, and consequently remained
long unprinted ; thus their fame was obscured, and
Guy of Chauliac got a quiet opportunity of appro-
priating no little of them.   The Church, to extend
a rigid frame for society as widely as possible, took
under its protection the Civil as well as the Canon
Law ; and in Medicine its clerks found, in the
galenist code, a congruous system of dogma.   But
with mordant raillery Henry declared that God did
not exhaust His creative power in making Galen ;
he twitted the clerks who were supposed to know
surgery by the grace of God, and asked how a man
is to make even so small a thing as a nail by listen-
ing to lectures on the art, or indeed by merely
watching others do it for ever so long.   As himself
a clerk, he reminds us of the well-known chapter in
the *Ethics* where we are told to learn virtue by the
practice of it ; as builders learn by building, and
harpers by playing the harp.   With Lanfranc he
insisted on anatomy as the foundation of Medicine ;
at Montpellier, where he had some relations with
Gordon the learned author of the *Lilium Medicinae*,
he taught anatomy by bones and pictures, as he had
learnt it at Bologna ; and he prefixed an anatomical
introduction to his *Surgery*, as Guy, Paré and others
did after him.   While declaring that too much faith in
books chokes natural talent, he resented almost with
violence the gibe that surgery is merely a handicraft;
if the mind must inform the hand in its operation,

the hand in its turn instructs the mind to interpret
the general proposition by the particular instance.
By experience without reason, he says, we make
some progress, but by reason without experience we
cannot get along at all.   He lashes the physicians
and counsels the students of his time with the
merciless wit of Petrarch, Rabelais or Molière, and
with the worldly wisdom of Polonius.   The poor
man's case every doctor tries to shuffle out of; the
high-born and rich, with their impatient changes of
doctors and their deficiency of ideas, are sketched
as vividly as if he had lived to-day : some of them
he says also " malentes in corporibus pati, quam in
bursa."   Yet after all his device to out-cunning the
cunning, and to out-cozen the cozeners, he says
well—" if you have operated conscientiously on
the rich for a proper fee, and on the poor for
charity, you need not play the monk, nor make
pilgrimages for your soul."

Into Paris then, in academical form such as we
have described it, Henry of Mondeville entered as,
for the most part, a loyal disciple of Lanfranc ; and
aided, as it would seem, by John Pitard,[1] Surgeon
to Philip the Fair, attempted for wounds to banish
Galen's salve surgery, and to introduce the new
methods of Hugh and Theodoric : for his pains he

[1] Jean Pitard or Pitart (Giovanni Pitardi), like Lanfranc, was
probably one of the Italian academic surgical physicians who to
the benefit of France were driven from Italy by wars and civil
commotion.   He was indeed one of those great physicians, like
Hugh of Lucca, whose radiance has persisted to our own day,
although no line of his writings, if ever he wrote any, survives.
By the College of St. Côme he was raised to an almost mythical
renown, as a reputed founder.

exposed himself to bad language, threats and perils; and, "had it not been for Truth and Charles of Valois," to far worse things. So he warns the young and poor surgeon not to plough the sand; but to prefer complaisance to truth, and ease to new ideas. I will summarise briefly the teaching of Mondeville on the cardinal features of the new method:—Wash the wound scrupulously from all foreign matter; use no probes, no tents—except under special circumstances; apply no oily or irritant matters; *avoid the formation of pus, which is not a stage of healing but a complication.* "Wounds dry much better before suppuration than after it." " Sequitur ergo minor probata quod in omni vulnere in quantum possumus evitare causas generationis saniei. Sequitur ulterius conclusio principalis quod possibile est omne vulnus in quantum hujusmodi sic procuratum curari absque eo quod fiat in eo notabilis generatio saniei." Theodoric had said before him " Sanies vulnus corrodet et auget." Henry then proceeds to combat those galenist doctrines which were contrary to his own experience, and proceeds thus:—Distinguish always between oozing hæmorrhage, hæmorrhage by jets, and that which pumps out of an inward wound; using styptics for oozing, and for jets the cautery or, where practicable, digital compression for not less than a full hour (*vide* p. 34). In another place he points out the fault of the cautery —that when the eschar falls the hæmorrhage may recur, and the wound must be disturbed for a second application. So for large vessels he advises acupressure, in these words:—" Infigatur acus cum filo sub utraque extremitate venae aut arteriae, et nectatur illud filum et fortiter stringatur." " But let the vessel be isolated from all surrounding parts with the knife, and torsion may be practised with ligature." His words are (Oportet) " scindere carnem exteriorem quae est supra extremitates venae aut arteriae e qua fluit sanguis, deinde dictas extremitates extrahere, torquere, et ligare." Lanfranc had given the warning not to let a nerve get caught in a ligature.[1] Henry proceeds—do not, as Galen teaches, allow the wound to bleed, with the notion of preventing inflammation ; for you will only weaken the patient's vitality (virtus), give him two diseases instead of one, and favour secondary hæmorrhage. When your dressings have been carefully made, do not interfere with them for some days ; keep the air out, for a wound left in contact with the air suppurates ; however, should pain and heat arise, open and wash out again, or even a poultice may be necessary ; but do not pull your dressings about, nature works better alone : if first intention fail she may succeed in the second, as a jeweller if he can solder gold to gold does so, if not, he has to take to borax ; these resources however we learn well not by arguing but by operating.[2] By the

[1] I have read a story somewhere in medieval surgical literature of a patient whose musculo-spiral nerve was thus caught and crushed by a surgeon while tying an artery of the arm. Thenceforth the wretched operator hardly dare show himself in the streets, for the patient would furiously pursue him, shaking the palsied arm and hurling execrations.

[2] The reader must understand the conviction was rooted in the medieval mind that the way to discover truth was by disputation.

new method you will have no stinks, shorter con-
valescence, and clean thin scars. In wounds of the
neck he says that alterations of the voice suggest
some implication of the larynx. When using the
word " Nature " he freely admits that the word is
an equivocal one; but he would speak of her alle-
gorically, as " a lute-player to whose melodies the
physician has to dance." Here he detaches himself
from medieval ontology (pp. 20 and 50) and returns
to that ministry of nature which was the key to the
Medicine of Hippocrates, and was renewed again in
Paré's admirable " Je l'ai pansay, Dieu le guarit."

To illustrate the care of this surgeon I will
quote also the following instructions :—" Always put
your needles and thread in order before you begin
to operate, and the thread not in a tangle, or you
will have to wait and rethread it; now blood will
not wait." He then describes an ingenious turn
—not a knot—of the thread, so that by one twitch
it will come straight away. Needles are to be of
various sizes, triangular and sharp, and *clean, or
they will infect the wound*; there must be grooves
by the sides of the eye into which the thread may
fall so as not to hurt as the flesh is pierced. The
processes of suture, a prolific source of controversy
and various practice in medieval surgery—as the
fear of access of air (p. 9), or of retention of
putrid matters had the ascendancy—are enjoined
with no less precision and foresight. If the
edges of a wound be altered by exposure they
must be refreshed. " If treated on Theodoric's
and my instructions, *every simple wound will heal*

without any notable quantity of pus." Every cause of
formation of pus is to be avoided, not only irritating
applications ("medicinae quae faciunt nasci pus,"
says Theodoric), but exposure, high diet, œdema, or
local plethora. "Many more surgeons know how
to cause suppuration than how to heal a wound."[1]

His caustic and reckless wit is manifest in his
remarks on the effects of the mind on the body.
If your patient is losing heart tell him he has been
nominated to a canonry : never mind whether your
story be true or untrue.

For the misfortune of Europe social progress is
discontinuous ; the civil faction fights of Italy in
the fourteenth century, the schism of the Papacy,
and a wave of mysticism, drew much of the life
from the universities of this gifted people, then
and in the fifteenth century so apt to engraft the
fruits of art upon the conceptions of learning.
Petrarch lamented the flagging of Salerno, Bologna,
and Padua. Boccaccio found the library of Monte
Cassino doorless, the grass growing on the window-
sills, and the books covered with filth. Bologna was
drooping in spite of Mundino, the father of modern
anatomy ; but as it drooped so Montpellier waxed.
In the thirteenth and fourteenth centuries, as I

[1] The copy of Henry of Mondeville I have chiefly used is in
old French, published by the Society of Old French Texts, edited
by Dr. A. Bos from the unique MS. of the Bibliothèque Nationale,
Paris, in 1897. But Henry being a clerk, wrote, what was probably the original copy of his *Surgery*, in latin. This first text
(from which I have quoted) was edited by Dr. Pagel in 1892. The
edition of Nicaise (Paris, 1893) is of course indispensable.

have said (p. 24), books were to a university what
the millionaire is, or ought to be, in the twentieth.
Montpellier, with Italy on the East and Cordova
on the West, became as rich in books as Paris
was poor.   Even in the later fourteenth century
there appear to have been only nine medical
works in the University of Paris; nor in the
fifteenth was it much richer until in 1498 Charles
VIII. carried off the library of St. Mark in
Florence, which contained some 800 MSS., and
Louis XII. that of Pavia; a transfer of books
which probably led to Brissot's venesection revolt in
1514 (p. 107).   But Montpellier had obtained all
Constantine's and Gerard's translations; Charles
of Anjou secured a copy of the *Continent* of Rhazes
—till then unknown in Europe; and one of her
elder sons—Arnold of Villanova (p. 32)—added to
Gerard's translations of Avicenna.   The *Surgery*
of Albucasis, chiefly derived from the Sixth Book
of Paul of Egina, and this in its turn from
Celsus and Galen, was of great assistance in the
early Middle Ages (p. 24), and handed on a
body of surgery to Lanfranc, Salicet, Henry of
Mondeville, and Guy of Chauliac.   Much of Galen
was at Montpellier; and, in the fourteenth century,
the Sixth, or Surgical Book of Paul of Egina itself,
afterwards to be lost again till the fifteenth.   On
the other hand Alexander of Tralles was no surgeon;
and the surgery of Hippocrates was only apprehended in the allusions of Galen.   The transcripts
of Aetius were as yet undiscovered, and the original
work of Celsus had been lost again.

Still Guy of Chauliac, who flourished in the second half of the fourteenth century, was enabled to feed his virile and inquisitive spirit on rich sources of learning. While he succeeded to the stores of Arnold and Gordon, with his just and cautious reason, and wealth of experience he cast out of them much of the sorcery, jugglery, astrology, and mysticism which were their reproach. Chauliac is a village in the Auvergne, and Guy was but a farmer's lad : it was by the aid of powerful friends that he studied at Toulouse and Montpellier, took orders, and the degree of Master of Medicine ; in his time there was no degree of Doctor of Medicine in France. Then he studied anatomy at Bologna under Bertruccio, the successor of Mundino—a study which, with Henry, he regarded as the foundation of surgery. The surgeon ignorant of anatomy, he says, " carves the human body as a blind man carves wood." Thence he paid a brief visit to Paris where for a moment, by the renown of Lanfranc, Jean Pitard, and Henry of Mondeville, surgery was in the ascendant. For the moment the Church and the Faculty had not succeeded in paralysing the scientific arm of Medicine. Guy began practice in Lyons, whence he was called to Avignon by Clement VI. as " venerabilis et circumspectus vir, dominus Guijo de Cauliaco, canonicus et praepositus ecclesiae Sancti Justi Lugduni, medicusque domini Nostri Pape." In Avignon he stayed, while other physicians fled, to minister to the victims of the plague (A.D. 1348), and he may have attended Laura, in spite of

Petrarch's tirades against all physicians, and even against Guy himself. His description of this epidemic is terrible in its naked simplicity. He did not indeed himself escape; he had an attack with bubo, and was ill for six weeks. He gave succour also in a later epidemic in Avignon, in 1360. His *Chirurgia Magna*, or *Inventarium seu Collectorium Artis chirurgicalis medicinae*— so called in distinction to the meagre little handbooks or *Chirurgiae Parvae* compiled from the larger treatises — was in preparation in 1363. This great work I have studied carefully,[1] and not without prejudice; yet I cannot wonder that Fallopius compared the author to Hippocrates, or that John Freind calls him the Prince of Surgeons. It is rich, aphoristic, orderly and precise. As a clerk, he wrote in latin, in the awkward hybrid tongue that medical latin then was, containing many Arabian, Provençal and French words, but very little greek [2] (p. 25).

The sects of surgery in his time Guy made to be five:—(1) Those who (like Galen and himself) promoted coction and suppuration; (2) those who, after Theodoric, taught the dry management of wounds with washings of wine; (3) those who, after Lanfranc and Salicet, trimmed, and used mild unguents and plasters; (4) those who used charms, with oil, wool, and cabbage leaves, and supposed God to have deposited His grace " in verbis, herbis

[1] Chiefly in the edition of Nicaise, Paris, 1890; incidentally in various editions in the Library of Cambridge University.

[2] The curious reader may be referred to the three editions of *Guidon en francoys* by Jehan Falcon, Dean and Professor of Montpellier, published 1520, 1534, and 1537.

et lapidibus "; (5) women and silly folk, who sat
and folded their hands under the will of God, Amen
—which may remind us of one of the happy sayings
of Henry that " the vulgar divide diseases into those
which have causes and those which have none."

That Guy should have emancipated himself from
the thraldom of authority is not to be expected;
no man of his day could look upon Aristotle with
an equal eye.   Yet the critical spirit of the great
southern surgeons was awake in him.   He scorned
the physicians of his day " who followed each other
like cranes, whether for love or fear he would not
say."   In courtesy and honour he showed a far
gentler and loftier temper than Henry; though
indeed it is hard to say when Henry is serious,
when ironical, and when medieval.   In respect of
its unity of reason and practice, Malgaigne con-
siders Guy's *Surgery* a masterpiece of learned and
luminous writing.   Guy was a more adventurous
surgeon than Lanfranc; as was indeed Franco, a
later Provençal, than Paré.   Guy still kept clear
of cutting for stone, as Paré did after him; but
Paré had the eminent example of Franco before his
eyes.   Guy did, however, operate for radical cure
of hernia, and for cataract; operations till his time
left wholly to the wayfaring specialists.

Nevertheless in respect of surgical principles, as
I have foreshadowed, Guy was not infallible.   Too
sedulous a disciple of galenism, he was as a deaf
adder to the new message of Hugh of Lucca, Theodoric and Henry; and not only was he deaf himself but, as the authoritative writer of the early

renaissance, he closed the ears of his brethren, even to
the day of Lister.   This is the more remarkable as
in Guy we find an historical sense, the first criticism
of medicine and medical authors on broad lines of
judgment, since Celsus.   If his judgments were not
always true they were always weighty.   Even
Haller never penned a more discriminating judgment
than this of Guy on Galen : " fuit enim maximus
in scientia demonstrativa " ; this on Albucasis also
is   notable : — " omnes   praedecessorum   suorum
majorum doctrinas congregavit, quas tamen non
elegit."   I regret to say his opinion of Gaddesden's
Rosa Anglicana—" una rosa fatua et sine odore
suavitatis "—is not to our credit.[1]   In respect of
the thesis I am supporting to-day, he says, " et
usque ad eum (Avicenna) omnes inveniuntur fuisse
physici et chirurgici.   Sed post, vel propter lassi-
viam vel occupationem curarum, nimium separata
fuit chirurgia et demissa in manus mechanicorum."
Guy was a man rather of sound judgment than
of penetrating insight.   Rich and comprehensive
as were his talents, he was not a man of genius
as we speak of genius in Lanfranc or William
Salicet ; nor had he the ardour or the audacity of
Henry.   At the close of his century he appears
rather as an equable, sensible and critical than an
inventive spirit.   As in the medieval schools, he
was disposed to balance his authorities—Avicenna,
Haly, Albucasis, Lanfranc, Theodoric, Salicet, Henry,
and so forth—by enumeration rather than by

[1] Dr. Payne says that Guy had in view John of Gaddesden, not
Gilbert (v. et Freind (2nd ed.) ii. 274).

appreciation.   Shrewd, and full of learning and experience, he lacked the fine temerity of the greatest
surgeons ; with all his sagacity he was prone to be too
judicious, too eclectic.   For instance, Yperman the
great fourteenth century surgeon of the Netherlands
(p. 35), divided scrofulous patients into those who
are touched by the king for the evil and those who
are not ; slily adding that some get well without
the touch, others are touched and do not get
well ; Guy on the other hand says sedately :—
" Concedo tamen quod virtute divina Serenissimus
Rex Franciae tangendo liberet multos."   Moreover
his influence, so long dominant, was, as I have said,
exercised against the true principles of the treatment of wounds.

Unfortunately also, we find reflections upon
surgeons of his own period which are harsh, unjust, and either ill informed or disingenuous.   On
the sense of literary honesty and magnanimity in
those times we can only hold our peace.   These
virtues were unbegotten.   Guy was a sinner ; but
even Paré sinned with him.

Of his substantial advances in surgery no sufficient account is possible ; but some chief points,
with the aid of Haeser, Malgaigne and Nicaise, I
may briefly sum up thus :—He pointed out the
dangers of surgery of the neck, among them that of
injuring the voice by section of the recurrent
laryngeal nerve, a precaution he probably learned
from Paul.   He urges a low diet for the wounded,
as did Mondeville and many others.   He uses sutures
well and discreetly (p. 9), but with far too many

E

salves.   On fractures of the skull he is at his best;
he notes the escape of cerebro-spinal fluid, and the
effect of pressure on the respiration.   It is somewhat strange that, in days of war, the study of chest
wounds had been rather neglected by Galen, Haly,
and Avicenna; their practice however was to leave
them open, lest pus should gather about the heart.
Theodoric and Henry ordered chest wounds to be
closed "lest the vital spirits escape."   Guy also
closed these wounds, unless there were any effusion
to be removed.   In empyema he objects to caustics,
and prefers the knife.   For hæmorrhages he used
sutures—a little too closely perhaps, styptics,
cautery, or ligature.   Sinuses he dilated with tents
of gentian root, or he incised them upon a director.
On ulcers his large experience is fully manifest; he
describes the carcinomatous kind as hopeless, unless
the mass can be excised at a very early stage and
the incision followed by caustics.   If in fractures and
dislocations he tells us nothing new, these sections
testify to a remarkable fulness of knowledge at a
period when the Hippocratic treatises were unknown.
Haeser says that in respect of position in fractured
femur he was the best physician of the Middle
Ages.   On the other hand my own reading tells
me that Guy restored and reanimated the vicious
doctrine that the healing of a wound is the work
of the surgeon; that not by natural process and
bodily function is it brought about—as Theodoric and Henry had taught—but by the educative
means of the surgeon operating upon a modifiable
entity (p. 20).   In it, it is the surgeon who models,

who incarnates, who builds; who commands the
elaborate methods and the recondite means—tents,
tampons, salves and plasters—by which these processes are initiated and governed; who assembles the
functions, engenders and regulates the new flesh,
and knits up the scar.

With Guy of Chauliac, the ablest surgeon of
his time, medieval medicine may be said to end.
The vigorous push of surgery in the thirteenth and
fourteenth centuries was checked in the West by
the feudal pride and academic bigotry which, cul-
minating in the reactionary ferocity of the Church,
thrust surgery down into the ranks of illiterate
barbers, reckless specialists, and adventurous charlatans.   In Italy, however, the genius and bent of
the people, for art as well as for philosophy, and
the ascendancy of the secular element in the
Universities, still kept surgery more nearly to its
place as the positive and fruitful side of Medicine,
and as "the scientific arm of the physician." [1]
Provence, strengthened for a time by the Arabs on
the south-west, by the Italians on the south-east,
and by the Papal Court at Avignon, had produced
Mondeville and Guy of Chauliac; and was to produce Franco.   But the slackness of the Italian
schools of medicine was temporary, as the advantages
of Montpellier were temporary.   In the fifteenth
century Bologna rose again quickly to surpass all
other schools, to surpass in vitality if not in

[1] An excellent phrase which I owe to Sir John Burdon Sanderson.

numbers Montpellier and even Paris. We have
seen that before the rich endowments of its chairs
Salerno, the oldest medical school of modern Europe,
had diminished. Moreover, as Paris waxed, Montpellier and Toulouse, Oxford and Cambridge,
stiffened under its harsh and sapless domination.
In spite of the Italians and Mondeville, Guy's
influence turned the tide back towards arabist and
galenical polypharmacy and salve surgery; and
turned it, not in France only but even in Italy
itself, where he influenced Argelata, and in Germany,
where he influenced Brunschwig (p. 91). During
the fifteenth and sixteenth centuries, fifty - two
editions of Guy's *Surgery* were printed; and it held
the field until tradition was broken again in Italy
by Fabricius, who founded surgery anew upon
anatomy and upon the original texts of Hippocrates,
Galen, Celsus and Paul, and fortified the new edifice
with the work of his own talents and experience
and those of his contemporaries, such as Fallopius
and Eustachius. Still in Italy of the fifteenth
century surgery never withered as it did in the
West; if it slumbered for a spell, it soon awoke
again, to be refreshed in the new hellenism.

Peter of Argelata (d. 1423), Doctor of Arts and
Medicine, and a professor of Bologna, wrote an
excellent *Surgery* full of personal observation; and,
perhaps for the first time, was frank about his own
mistakes. In some bolder adventure in operative
work, as distinguished from mere wound-surgery,
Peter followed the lead of Henry and Guy; and was
himself a learned and skilful practitioner. He was

for a dry wound; but to this end used powders which, as we have seen, Hugh and Theodoric refused, as retentive of putrescent matters. He helped himself freely of course to Guy's writings, but was bold in preferring experience to authority. He used sutures for the larger wounds, with drainage tubes of perforated metal. He trepanned the long bones as well as the skull, and even operated in the lines of the specialists on hernia and stone. He cured fistula by incision, and in extraction of the dead fœtus followed Guy's method of operating through a large spectrum.

Of one of Peter's pupils, Marcello Cumano, a surgeon known to few of us even by name, I must speak in passing; for, if De Renzi be correct, he was the first to write upon the wounds of firearms. Cumano was an army surgeon who died in the Morea, and the manuscript of his *Vade Mecum* lay unknown in Florence till 1650. It was printed not " eighteen " years later, but seventeen. I cannot discover the grounds of Haeser's commendation of this surgeon. The edition [1] which I had before me as I wrote this paragraph is but a " Chirurgia parva," a meagre collection of galenical receipts, many of them, it is important to note, for venereal eruptions; I discover not a gleam in it of surgical or medical sagacity. His writing on shot wounds is exiguous, even as a beginning. This paragraph is entitled *Dolor vulneris sclopeto illati vel ballista.* The pain is to be soothed by the warm application

[1] A collection of medical tracts published at Ulm. Ed. Velschius, 1667.

of oil of roses, of galbanum and of assafœtida.
This receipt does not suggest that the opinion was
then current that these wounds were poisoned; but
the author does not discuss the matter, as Haeser
seems to imply. The discovery of firearms shook
not the nations only, but also the dominion of
authority in Medicine, by raising, as we shall
presently see, another and a new controversy on
the treatment of wounds.

Leonardo Bertapaglia, another great Paduan
Professor, flourished a little after Peter of Argelata,
but was a man of far less originality. He held
more closely to the Arabs, especially to Avicenna
and salve surgery; he knew but little anatomy,
and not only, like other wound surgeons, avoided
major operations, but left even minor operations to
the barbers, wherein he betrayed the weakness
which had crept even into the surgery of the
Universities of harassed Italy. Moreover we note
in his *Surgery* the advancing influence of Arabian
astrology in this century. Still, Bertapaglia did
good service in investigating the conditions and
improving the method of the ligature. His method
was to draw the vessel forwards with a steel hook,
to isolate it, to tie it with a flaxen thread, then, to
prevent slipping, to pierce it with the needle and
thread and, twisting the thread round, to make
fast by knots. It was a clumsy method, but in
isolation of the vessel was better than Paré's *ligature
en masse*. He resected ribs in empyema, as Guy
had done; he sutured wounds of the intestine,
with the glover's ("furrier's") stitch, and used

softened catgut in preference to thread for the purpose.

At Padua, in the fifteenth century, by the hand of Montagnana the elder, were instituted the *Consilia,* or published collections of notes and reflections on cases, which played so efficient a part in the advance of clinical Medicine in the two following centuries. For Montagnana we cannot claim more than a commencement, yet he also was among the first of those who returned to the fountains of Greek. He quotes directly from Paul, whose writings had disappeared for a while after Guy used them; and from Celsus, whose great work had been recovered again, in 1443, in the church of St. Ambrose at Milan (p. 25 n.).

In the midst of these mainly arabist professors of Medicine of the fifteenth century arose Antonio Benivieni, to be revered as the forerunner of Morgagni, and as one of the greatest physicians of the late Middle Ages. This distinguished man, a Doctor of Medicine and a man of culture, was born in 1448 and died in 1502. He was not a professor but an eminent practitioner in Florence, at a period when, in spite of its platonism (p. 63), Florence on the whole was doing the most for science; for as Bologna turned to law Padua turned to humanism and philosophy. He was one of those fresh and independent observers who, like Mondeville, was oppressed by the authority neither of Arab nor Greek. Malgaigne claims for him the first performance of lithotrity; but even if this statement were correct,[1] Benivieni's case

[1] Lithotrity, or lithothripsy, is an old story. Attempts at it were made by Byzantines and Arabs, more or less as secrets of the

was in a woman, in whom the stone was hooked
forward, and then knocked to bits with a punch.[1]
Carefully as the bits were washed out, this operation in woman, even if it had not been anticipated,
was no great matter in lithotrity. Nor do his claims
to our admiration rest upon his puncture of the
hymen for retained menses ; nor upon his division
and slow extension of the cicatricial contractions
of a burned arm, ingenious as these devices were.
Nor again shall we admire Benivieni chiefly
because he was the first to communicate his own
matter tersely and practically, without fabricating
a complete treatise to contain it, and without
tricking it out with dogmatisings, ratiocination, or
the chimeras of oriental lore. This is true enough,
no doubt; but Malgaigne does not state that

adept. A remarkable passage from the *Corpus script. hist.
Byzant.* (vol. ii. p. xxxiv.) is quoted by Haeser (Bk. i. p. 509)
(I paraphrase the Greek, but keep closely to the meaning) :—
*In one afflicted with a very chronic dysuria instruments were passed
by the natural passage* (τοῦ φυσικοῦ ὑπονόμου) *into the bladder,
which breaking up* [*the stones*] (διαθρύπτοντα) *promoted their
discharge and thus gave free issue to the urine.* Haller points
out that a later surgeon, Sanctorius (*Comm. Avicennae*, 1626),
pictured a trifid catheter with a spear in it, wherewith to pierce
the stone, but regards it as a mere suggestion. In a MS. at
Vercelli however Haeser says a long pair of nippers is figured
with such a boring stem, the instrument to be passed *per
urethram.* Ciucci of Arezzo and Rome (about 1650) invented such
an instrument—very like that of Civiale ; and says by its means his
own bladder was relieved of a stone in three sittings. He adds
that the bladder may be caught in the nippers and torn, when (the
operator) "misero patienti et lapidem et animam educit ! " In his
own case he laid upon the operator " ut mihi religiosissime obtem-
perasset," and that if he felt the least catch on the bladder the
operator should stop instantly.

[1] Celsus tells us that the Alexandrine surgeon Ammonius
(ὁ λιθότομος) used the same means, in both sexes, to break up stones
too large to pass by the perineal incision. (Lib. vii. ch. 26, § 3.
Védrène's Ed. p. 540.)

the little book *De abditis causis morborum* (brief
title) was not published in any form by Antony
Benivieni himself, but posthumously by his brother
Jerome, who found these precious notes in Antony's
desk after his death, and with the cordial consent
of a friend,[1] competent in the subject, published
them in 1506,[2] in the form which no doubt justly
merits our admiration.   Benivieni's chief fame for
us is far more than all this; it is that he was the
founder of pathological anatomy.   So far as I know
he was the first to make the custom and to declare
the need of necropsy to reveal what he called not
exactly " the secret causes " but the hidden causes
of diseases.   Before Vesalius, before Eustachius, he
opened the bodies of the dead as deliberately and
clear-sightedly as any pathologist in the spacious
times of Baillie, Bright, and Addison.   Virchow, in
his address at Rome, said Morgagni was the first
pathologist who, instead of asking What is disease ?
asked Where is it ?   But Benivieni asked this
question plainly before Morgagni : not only, says
he, must we observe the disease but also with more
diligence search out the seat of it.   The precept is
so important I will quote the original words :—
"*Oportet igitur medicum non solum morbum cognoscere,
sed et locum in quo fit, diligentius perscrutari.*"
Among his pathological reports are morbus coxae
(two cases) ; biliary calculus (two cases) ; abscess of

[1] Rosalius, who says that the loss of such notes "magnum
detrimentum, magna injuria fieret cum presentis tum futuri saeculi
hominibus."

[2] The R.C.P.L. copy—a pretty one, containing *Scribonius Largus*
also, was printed by Cratander of Basil in 1529.

the mesentery; thrombosis of the mesenteric vessels; stenosis of the intestine; some remarkable cardiac cases, several of " polypus " (clot, which was a will-of-the-wisp to the elder pathologists); scirrhus of the pylorus, and probably another case in the colon; ruptured bowel (two cases); caries of ribs with exposure of the heart (*vide* Galen's case, p. 17). He gives a good description of senile gangrene which even Paré did not discriminate. He seems to have had remarkable success in obtaining necropsies : concerning one fatal case he says plaintively " Sed nescio qua superstitione versi negantibus cognatis," etc. Of another he says " cadavere publicae utilitatis gratia inciso " (the case of cancer of the stomach).[1] With this admirable and original leader Italian Medicine of the fifteenth century closes gloriously, to slumber for some fifty years, till the dayspring of the new learning. Of his work Malgaigne says, and apparently with truth, that " up to now it is the only work on pathology which owes nothing to any one."[2]

Some of my readers may wonder how it is that

[1] It is interesting to note that Benivieni held the opinion of the march of the " French Pox," that it was from Spain to Italy, and from Italy to France. The pestilence seems to have received this name on the invasion of Naples by the French in 1495. The note on Benivieni as a pathologist in Signor Chiari's " History of Pathological Anatomy " in the second volume of Puschmann's *Handbuch*, seems to me very inadequate to the proper appreciation of his merits.

[2] Dodoens published an edition of Benivieni at Leyden in 1585, with notes of his own, which has not fallen in my way. Nor have I seen the fifty additional records discovered in the last century, and published by Puccinotti (see Haeser *in loc.*). Haeser tells us that we have to lament the loss of a work of Benivieni on Surgery. He says that for hæmorrhage he used the cautery "*incisam arteriam candente ferro inuro.*"

in discoursing of medieval surgery I have not dwelt upon the surgical College of St. Côme of Paris. Well, St. Côme did no great things for surgery. The truth is that, infected with the exclusiveness and dialectical conceits of all the schools of Paris, St. Côme was almost ready to sacrifice surgery itself if thereby it might choke off its parasites the barbers. Lest they should be suspected of mixing their philosophy with facts, its members went about with their hands ostentatiously tied behind them. If perhaps Malgaigne speaks too contemptuously of St. Côme, it must be admitted that the College was in a false position throughout. In aping the Faculty of Medicine, it lost touch of mother earth without gaining any harbourage in the deep waters of the proud. Nay, such is the Nemesis of pride, the barbers came to command the position. It did not suit the Faculty to see the barbers weakened; for in their weakness lay the strength of the surgeons of St. Côme, who sought incessantly to appear as lettered clerks, to attach their College to the University, and even to claim a place beside the Faculty itself. To bring St. Côme to its knees, and to check the presumptuous claims of this Corporation on the privileges of the Faculty of Medicine, on a liberal education in arts and medicine, on a place in the university, on the suppression of unqualified surgical practice, and, less honourably, on relief from handicraft and urgent calls,[1] the Faculty had but to coquette with

---

[1] To be subject to urgent calls was in the opinion of the time the status of a slave. I trust that none of my readers can see any excuse for such a sentiment.

the barbers. Medicine, proclaimed the Faculty
when it suited its purpose, contains the theoretical
and the practical sides of surgery ; a surgeon is
therefore but the servant of the physician. If
St. Côme sought to provide lectures in surgery,
the Faculty, which kept possession of teaching
licenses and desired in the surgeon a docile
assistant, took the teaching from the college,
and invited the barbers to lectures of its own. In
their duplicity and conceit of caste physicians of
the Faculty condescended even to publish books on
surgery, books as arid and as insincere as their
lectures. On the other hand, in the person of the
King's Barber, the barbers had a secret and potent
influence at Court.[1] The Faculty persisted in
denying to St. Côme all " esoteric " teaching, all
diagnosis, and all use of medical therapeutics.
Aristotle was pronounced to be unfavourable to
the " vulgarising of science." Joubert was attacked
for editing Guy, but replied with dignity (in the
notes to his edition). While the Faculty thus tried
to prevent the access to letters of a presumptuous
body of artisans, St. Côme in mimic arrogance
disdained the barbers, sought to deny them the
name of surgeon, and was jealous of the diffusion
of technical knowledge among them in the vernacular tongue.[2] Thus, as it was only during the

[1] In 1372 the Barbers obtained the right "de curir et de guérir
toutes manières de clous, bosses, apostumes, et plaies ouvertes en
cas de péril, et autrement si les plaies n'étaient mortelles, sans
pouvoir en estre empêchés par les mires, ou chirurgiens jurés." At
Hildesheim at any rate the Barbers dedicated their guild (1487) to
St. Côme and Damian (Becker, *loc. cit.* p. 29, n. 3).
[2] Tolet in his translation of Paul of Egina into latin (Lyons,

brief ascendancy of the great southern surgeons, such as Lanfranc, Pitard, and Henry of Mondeville, who were both surgeons and scholars, that St. Côme exercised any real and beneficial influence, I have not occupied myself with this College at any greater length.

In discussing French surgery of the fifteenth century we must distinguish then between the surgery of Paris, of the provinces, and of the rural districts. And it would be unjust to forget that in the latter half of the fifteenth century Paris suffered some reforms, although the public was then as convinced that orders were essential in a physician as now in a schoolmaster; celibacy was abolished for physicians, and with it diminished the allurements of prebends and rectories, and the pernicious practice of the "médecins reclus" (Buchärzte) who did not visit patients, nor even see them, but received their ambassadors, who brought gifts and vessels of urine, and carried back answers far more presumptuous than the wise response of Falstaff's physician.[1] Nevertheless reform in Paris was not only very grudging, but was capriciously favoured or thwarted by the Court. Fortunately however the surgeons were carried out of Paris into war, a far better school than the barren Faculty of Medicine.

1540) says he was not disposed to let the surgeons learn latin, as this would be to rival the physicians in knowledge "ce que les médecins ne doivent vouloir."

[1] In the many handbooks of the water casters to be found in our libraries are schedules of the colours and other superficial appearances of the urine with the proper medicines in a parallel column.

Montpellier towards the end of the fifteenth and in the sixteenth century fell upon evil days. Deserted by the Popes who had maintained the liberal traditions of Italy, ravaged by war, and her libraries rifled, it was a sign as well as a cause of farther decay that, to herself untrue, she fell under the influence of Paris, and committed the fatal error of separating surgery farther from medicine, whereby she cut Medicine away from its living root, forbad her graduates even to meddle with the craft, and abolished surgical teaching.

Meanwhile, however, the return of the Popes to Rome, and the displacement of Albucasis and Avicenna by the greek texts, renewed the shrivelling body of Medicine, and with the help of anatomy Italian Medicine awoke again ; though until the days of Vesalius and Harvey the renascence came rather of men of letters than of medicine. The Arabs and Paris said ;—Why dissect if you trust Galen ? But the Italian physicians insisted on verification ; and therefore back to Italy again the earnest and clear-sighted students flocked from all regions. Vesalius was a young man when he professed in Padua, yet, young or venerable, where but in Italy would he have won, I will not say renown but even sufferance ! If normal anatomy was not directly a reformer of Medicine, by way of anatomy came morbid anatomy, as conceived by the genius of Benivieni, of Morgagni, and of Valsalva ; the galenical or humoral doctrine of pathology was sapped, and soaring in excelsis for the essence of disease gave place to grubbing for its roots.

We cannot make however brief an adventure on the history of Medicine in the sixteenth century, that dramatic century as vast and swift in the compass of its art and thought as bigoted and fierce in its reactions, without a livelier sense of that intimate dependence of Medicine upon the spirit of its age which we have recognised already. Tormented by pestilence and war, seeking a false succour in the black arts of the East, in astrology, magic, and priestcraft, our fathers of the sixteenth century fought a dark and troublous way to light, truth, and beauty. Amid materialism, indifference, and bold unbelief in Church and State, when even priests were making a mock of religion, it was the men of science, in the armour of natural knowledge, who awakened religion anew, and brought refreshment to stunted souls and withered hearts.[1] The platonism of this century, soon as it settled down on its lees, was for a while the powerful adversary of aristotelian orthodoxy, in cloister, in academy, and even in the Papal Chair. Da Vinci, Michael Angelo, Raphael, were Platonists; though, like Telesio who turned from the Church to natural philosophy, they rejected much of its flummery. Before them Petrarch had denounced inordinately, but he had given no lead. Vives, the Spanish Professor of Oxford and friend of Erasmus, was the first of a great procession of builders—De la Ramée, Palissy, Bacon, Charron, Gassendi, Descartes—who doomed the fabric of the dogmatic schools, and in letters and natural philosophy laid the stronger foundation of inductive

[1] For this true and profound reflection I am indebted to Haeser.

research.   Vives urged the study of anatomy, and
with De La Ramée (both of them laymen) declared
the futility of lectures on Medicine without clinical
instruction.   Such instruction was established in
Padua—by Montanus, and probably in Montpellier.
Paracelsus, as ardent a system-maker as Galen, in-
toxicated by platonism and blinded by an impatient
temper, did much service nevertheless in blowing
his horn over against the ancient and toppling
walls of convention ;   and, although he ignored
anatomy, he sketched in some chemical background
for Medicine.   The great princes of Florence, Milan,
Ferrara, and Mantua endowed liberal learning.
More than a century before Battista Porta in
Naples, and two centuries before Boyle and Wren
in Oxford, Bessarion in Rome, Pomponius Laetus
in Naples, Nicholas of Cusa in Germany had promoted associations of learned men which, directly and
indirectly, were the strength of science in successive
generations.   In the sixteenth century Palissy
founded the science of geology, a foundation scarcely
built upon till the nineteenth.   Bacon contrasted
the " anticipatio," or speculative conception of nature
—which he calls a rash and precocious method—
with the interpretation of nature ;   the logic of
thought being perfect enough he proclaimed that
the stuff and premises of it must be verified,
and that experiment must not be desultory, but
systematic and consistent ("seriatim et continenter").
Strangely lacking in the qualities of an investigator,
and too violent in reaction against hypothesis, yet
as a philosopher he inscribed on a monumental

page principles which Copernicus, Kepler, Galileo, Harvey, were putting into practice. Vesalius regenerated anatomy, by proving that Galen's anatomy was largely based upon dissection of apes and dogs, and in any case was faulty and defective.[1]   In physiology Colombo and Cesalpini were preparing for Harvey.   But ratiocination founded on scholastic dogmas is not upset in a year, nor in a century of years.   A ruthless war against enlightenment lasted all the second moiety of the sixteenth century, and well on into the seventeenth; for, as Hippocrates warned us, experience is difficult, verification fallible, observation long and costly, occasion fleeting.   Many changes however conspired to disturb the serenity of medical self-satisfaction, and to undermine the long domination of traditional medical doctrine which, even if genuine, would as a formal and transcendent authority have become sterile enough, and, as a bogus doctrine of partial and distorted texts, was infinitely mischievous.   Now however " uralte Wasser steigen verjüngst."   On the discovery of the original greek texts, the false texts, glosses and commentaries were put to shame ; while the invention of hempen or rag papers in place of silk paper or parchment, the discovery of printing, and the vindication of the vernacular tongues sapped the privileges of the clerks.

I have said elsewhere,[2] that the aid of the

---

[1] The *De corporis humani fabrica Libri septem* appeared in the same year (1543) as the *De revolutionibus orbium celestium*.

[2] *Harveian Oration* 1900.

humanists in the development of Medicine was no unmixed advantage; for if in art and letters they were reformers they were for the most part as scornful of handiwork, and as alien from natural knowledge, as the clerks and the nobles. It is true nevertheless that such men as Vidus Vidius— Francis the First's Regius Professor at the College of France—if themselves no very original observers, by leading their pupils back to the ancient texts, indirectly loosened the rusty chains of the galeno-arabist bondage, and of all such bondage; and in this work Vidius had successors greater than himself—such scientific humanists as Beroaldo of Bologna, Leoniceno of Ferrara, Linacre, Caius, and the two editors of the Hippocratic Canon, Cornarus and Foesius. From Petrarch to Molière great laymen had demanded why, if medicine were not a going concern, but a static doctrinal scheme derived, like the Athanasian Confession, from the fathers, and immutable, it needed any augurs, adepts, or illuminati for its comprehension and use. To this question there was no good answer; and thoughtful physicians influenced, perhaps insensibly, by the searching spirit of the greek texts of Hippocrates, began to stir in their sleep, and uneasily to suspect there were many maladies on which even this great ancient threw but a glimmering light or none,—such, for example, as syphilis and the great pestilences of the West, upon which new problems books began to appear, such as those of Fracastoro, Caius, and Baillou. Dialectical and scholastic as it was, Baillou's treatise made its mark as the first comprehensive treatise on Epidemics since Hippocrates ; in spite of himself he was compelled to teach what Galen did not know, to begin to discriminate certain fevers hitherto confounded under one name, and thus to develop symptomatology, and slowly and insensibly to bring into view authorities concurrent with the ancients themselves.

Other direct causes of the break-up of the frost were the use of firearms,[1] which made wounds that even Galen had failed to foresee or to provide against; a like defect of galenical doctrine in respect of syphilis and other epidemics ; not defect only but grievous error in anatomy ; the reform of this science ; the germination of pathological anatomy ; the prodigious discovery of a vast continent of which the omniscient ancients had no suspicion ; a strange schism on venesection—whether, that is, it were orthodox to bleed on the side of the disease or on the opposite side (p. 107) ; and the revelation in the light of the genuine Hippocratic treatises of the incompetence of the Arabs in fractures and luxations.[2]

In the opening of the century Italian Medicine was still in the van until the birth of the great French surgeons, Franco and Paré ; and of Gersdorff

[1] Although for siege work pieces of ordnance were used in the middle of the fourteenth century, field pieces and the small firearms did not come into use till a hundred years later.   The first picture of a cannon is in an illuminated MS. of the fourteenth century in the Christchurch Library.

[2] The chief Greek texts were not directly accessible till towards the middle and end of the sixteenth century ; but Aetius was discovered, and Celsus and Paul, more than once lost, were found again (pp. 25, note, and 55).

and Würtz in Germany. Among the great Italians
of this time, first perhaps in interest was the un-
lucky Berengario da Carpi, a pioneer in anatomy—
he tells us he had "dissected" a hundred bodies [1]
—and a Doctor of Medicine of Bologna, whose name
has been made familiar to us by Cellini. Cellini
maliciously twits Berengario on the enormous profits
of his practice in the French pox ; this he treated
by mercurial inunctions. Cardinal Colonna, well
known to us by his portrait by Raphael in the Uffizi,
was one of his most lucrative patients. Berengar
practised in Rome in the first part of the sixteenth
century. Twice he extirpated the uterus for pro-
lapsus ; he wrote an able treatise on gunshot
wounds ; and in the course of his anatomical inves-
tigations he added a few facts to pathology. A
still more celebrated physician was John of Vigo
(1460-1520) who, as attached to that fighting
Pope Julius II., saw much of field surgery. His
Surgery, printed at Rome 1514, had enormous
vogue, a vogue perhaps unique. If of Guy's
Surgery, at the end of the fifteenth century and
the beginning of the sixteenth, there were, as we
have seen, 52 editions, the run of editions and
translations of Vigo seems to have been endless.

[1] It is not easy to know what in those days "dissection of a
body" meant. The corpses soon became putrid, and on many
occasions probably a public demonstration of the chief viscera
sufficed. Moreover some of the bodies were probably of monkeys,
or only of the domestic pig, so useful to medieval anatomists. That
Berengar was an ardent anatomist however, even of the human
subject, may be confirmed from the persecutions he suffered at
the hands of the priests. Nevertheless all the anatomists before
Vesalius professed to work only in the illustration and elaboration
of Galen.

For since the work of Guy no standard surgical treatise had appeared.   A French translation of Vigo's treatise on the wounds of firearms fell into the hands of Paré, and probably, as a modern and independent work, had, with Guy's *Surgery*, then the standard authority, an inspiring influence upon the barber's boy while he was shaving, trimming wigs, or brushing out the shop at cockcrow.   Nevertheless the value of Vigo's work is far less ; he may be called the last of the elder or didactic surgeons, he had little of the initiative of Fabricius, and drew freely on Guy.   Yet he was a shrewd and skilful as well as a learned physician, who had read his Celsus to some profit.   In his *Practica,* published at Rome in 1514, he observed that gangrene is apt to arise from bad bandaging in fractures, and from access of frost ; also he compared wound gangrene with the dry senile form which, as I have said, had been described by Benivieni (p. 58) ; he noted fracture of the inner table of the skull without that of the outer ; and he undertook certain of the graver operations, though not such as fell within the custom of the professional cutters—not, that is to say, hernia, stone, plastic work, or cataract : these he discreetly left to the " vagabonds qui courent de pais en pais." He treated syphilis with mercurial inunctions. In amputation, like Benivieni, he relied upon the cautery, and mentions ligature only in the case of tying an uncut vessel before dividing it, as for example Antyllus did in aneurysm.   The current fame of Vigo is that he first wrote of the wounds of firearms, though a bare priority is said to belong to Cumano (p. 53). In respect of a controversy of which I shall have to speak more fully, John of Vigo held that the wounds of firearms were scorched and poisoned wounds, and therefore to be purified by the cautery and injections of boiling oil.

Although even in Italy pus kept in favour with physicians and surgeons alike, till Lister swept it away,[1] yet in the sixteenth century, as in all periods of the history of Medicine, surgery, being conversant directly with nature and fact, was before inner medicine to receive the inspiration of the new methods of personal experience and free inquiry. Indeed the unscholarly training of its practitioners saved them from the tyranny of the letter; while the enlightenment of truth slowly compelled the regard of their haughtier fellows. In all countries, Italy excepted where from Salernitan times onwards scientific surgery had always been held in honour, the barbers, the bone-setters and the cutters, the most intimate of the servants of nature, gained upon the superior surgical persons of the colleges, and demanded admission to their ranks. All honour to them; for these humble and faithful ministers of such medicine as they knew, tended the lepers and the syphilitic, and in times of pestilence stuck bravely to their posts when their

[1] Professor Howard Marsh makes the following note on this sentence:—"I do not think surgeons down to Lister (say Lawrence, Brodie, Paget or Syme) favoured, or, consciously, took steps to procure pus. But, not seeing how to avoid it, they desired 'healthy pus,' 'pus laudabile' instead of sanious or ichorous pus. They were always glad (even if surprised) when none formed."

betters stood timorously aloof, or even took to flight.

When we turn from these general considerations to consider the life of Franco, the surgeon who shares with Paré the glories of French Medicine of the sixteenth century, we shall see how it was from the depths not from the heights that Medicine was fed; from the springs not from the sky, which was as brass. There is a well-known passage in the Oath of Hippocrates, a passage well known not only as a part of that great injunction, but also as a somewhat unintelligible part : that, namely, in which the aspirant is to promise that he will not cut for stone, but will leave this operation to a peculiar class of practitioners. That this warning signifies surgery to be a calling inferior to medicine is, as Littré well says, an opinion devoid of the smallest probability, one which is belied by the whole of the Canon wherein the Greek physicians appear constantly as practitioners of medicine and surgery alike. And in so high a discourse it is difficult to accept the explanation of Franco that the counsel was one of vulgar prudence ; that Hippocrates, and after him Galen, not despising either the work or the workmen, yet shirked undertakings which were full of risk and exposed the surgeon to calumnious tongues. Franco murmurs indeed that if a patient die under medicine the faults of the physician are laid to the score of the imperfection of nature ; but that if he die under operation the surgeon is an executioner or a murderer, and not rarely has to take to his heels. Such are the words of the boldest of the responsible surgeons of the sixteenth century. Franco, like Paré, was no clerk; he came of a class lower even than that of Paré and the barbers, that class, mostly wanderers, of bonesetters, oculists, plastic operators, and cutters for stone and hernia, of whom I have often spoken. Seeing that until the time of Gersdorff and Paré the regular surgeons, if they ventured at all upon the larger amputations, postponed them till, to the certain witness of the bystanders, the patient was moribund, we cannot wonder that, even from the time of Hippocrates — to say nothing of the Egyptians — the dangerous ventral operations, and those on the eye which but too often were swiftly disastrous, fell into the hands of peripatetic craftsmen, runagates Gale calls them, men usually of low origin, ignorant, reckless, and rapacious. These travelling surgeons of the short robe operated but too often with great brutality,—and usually got out of reach before the issue. If the issue were fatal, or indeed without substantial relief to the patient, they stood a good chance of paying with their skins. In Dr. Henri-Maxime Ferrari's interesting book *Une Chaire de Médecine au XVme siècle* are some anecdotes of these operators, and of their mode of life. One of them, who by an operation on the eye had failed to relieve the pain of a certain lady (who would seem to have had a glaucoma?), was pursued in the night by her infuriated husband with a naked sword in his hand.

As the truss was a very clumsy instrument, at any rate till the end of the seventeenth century,

the radical cure of hernia was in great demand.[1]
In the district of Crotona twenty-seven families of
these special operators flourished for a long period.
In later times they got more culture, did substantial work for Medicine, and were called to
great nobles even down to the eighteenth century.[2]
One of them was surgeon to Sixtus IV. in Rome,
and to Francesco Sforza in Milan. But from the
time of Franco no important book came again from
such operators till that of Durante Scacchi of
Urbino in 1596. That Calabria was a chief
nursery of these cutters may possibly signify that
the craft had survived from the days of the Greek[3]
" Periodeutes " who pretty surely travelled to the
Doric Hellenes of Magna Graecia.[4] Now it is
the chief merit of Franco that he brought these
operations within the lines of responsible surgery,
raised them again to the standard of Celsus, and
thrust them into the ken of Paré and Fabricius.

The illustrious Provençal surgeon — " ce beau
génie chirurgical," as Malgaigne, in declining the
task of entering upon so full a life, calls Franco,—
was born about 1503. It is a note of his fearless
and penetrating spirit that he was a Huguenot, and

[1] So far as I remember Franco never even mentions the
truss. Fabricius of Hilden (p. 97) was perhaps the first surgeon
to bring the instrument into a practicable form.

[2] Cf. Fabbri's *History of the Lithotomists and Oculists of Norcia.*
Bologna, 1870.

[3] Of operation for hernia we have no record in the Hippocratic
canon ; if Praxagoras of Cos performed it (cf. *Caelius Aurelianus,*
Acut. morb. iii. 17) unfortunately the texts are not convincing.

[4] It is difficult here to avoid a passing allusion to the survival
of some precious rivulets of Greek art and Greek language which
had not dried up in Calabria in the time of the Pisani.

for his religious opinions was driven to Switzerland.[1] We may wish we had his concise opinion of the mock St. Côme, founded at Toulouse in 1517, whose "mires" (myrrhes) or "médecins chirurgiens," determined not to be behind the Paris body, declared "qu'il n'y avait rien de plus vil que la chirurgie," a "rifiuto" which the students joyfully acclaimed.

Franco began as an apprentice to an operating barber, and to a hernia specialist. He had no more "education" than Paré or Würtz, and he was spared the misfortune of a speculative intellect. Dr. Alezais[2] describes him as a "membre de St. Côme à Paris," but this is certainly incorrect. He picked up some anatomy, educated himself by observation, experience and manipulation, and as a simple operator or "Master" won considerable renown. As upright and modest as Paré, though he never attained Paré's social position, he submitted to work under the physicians, taking his quiet revenge in the remark that they did not know enough to distinguish good surgery from bad. Nicaise[3] says roundly "No surgeon made such discoveries as Franco; for hernia, stone and cataract he did much more than Paré." In comparison with Paré Haeser treats Franco somewhat slightingly, for not only did Franco bring the operations for hernia (whether for strangulation or for radical cure), lithotomy, diseases of the eye,

---

[1] The Waldensian massacres took place in 1545.

[2] *Les anciens Chirurgiens et Barbiers de Marseilles*, 1901.

[3] No longer do I write *Mons.* Nicaise, as unhappily this able historian at the height of his attainments has been taken from us.

and plastic operations into the field of legitimate
Medicine, but by the great advances he made in
the technique of these several departments he did
so with great effect.   In asserting that no surgeon
made more advances than Franco, and few so many,
Nicaise is probably right.   His compatriot of
Chauliac had much influence upon him, but
Guy had not made much adventure into these
specialist fields of surgery ; he had not in-
vaded the monopolies of the " vagabonds," nor
contended against their ignorance and audacity.
Whether from sheer ignorance, or the brutality of
habit, it had been the custom during the Middle
Ages, and down even till the middle of the seventeenth century, in operating for hernia—and in
spite of Celsus' clear distinction (vii. 21), hydrocele
and sarcocele were not too carefully discriminated
from hernia—to sacrifice one or even both testicles ;
an abuse against which Franco took successful precautions, and proved that the canal could be closed
and the ring sutured without castration.   In irre-
ducible inguinal hernia he distinguished between
opening and not opening the sac, and described
adhesions of sac and intestine.   From him indeed
dates the rational operation for strangulated hernia,[1]
and in strangulated scrotal hernia he founded the
method.   Paré, and after him Petit, condemned the

---

[1] The earlier practice of the specialists was to puncture the skin
and bowel, and after recession to apply the cautery to the skin.
Guy saw 30 cases so treated.   Fabricius inverted the patient
and shook him by the legs.   We must judge gently of such primi-
tive methods as these ; even Paré spoke favourably of reducing
hernia by strewing iron filings on the tumour, and administering
lodestone internally.

ablation of the testicle,[1] a procedure however which many surgeons thought quite good enough for priests; and for these advances he gives credit to Franco, though Fabricius does not even mention them.   But Paré did not himself attempt such operations ; he did the best he could with long recumbency, and the local use of bandages, plasters, strong astringents (such as dragons' blood), or cauterising and cicatrising agents.   In children it seems that, with the help of nature, such methods were not altogether fruitless ; but in spite of the improvement in trusses by both the surgeons distinguished under the name of Fabricius [2] and by later surgeons, the Council of Zurich even so late as 1693 had to forbid excision of the testicle, and indeed all herniotomy save in urgent cases.

Stone must have been a very common disease in the Middle Ages ; and cutting for stone, though surrendered to specialists, was in rather better hands than herniotomy ; for in large part, as I have said, it became the profession of responsible families of which the Collots, whose dexterity Paré commended, were the chief.   These men were not all charlatans by any means,[3] and in their hands no doubt the

[1] As Franco's book on hernia was published under the approval of the Chirurgiens-jurés of Paris and in two editions, Paré must have known it well.

[2] Fabrizio carried Paré's improvement of trusses so far forward that he reduced the operations of one Italian family of hernia cutters from 200 to 20 in the year.   Very early in the sixteenth century Benedetti, a Professor of Perugia, adopted a Spanish method of saving the testicle. (See Fabbri's history of these specialists.   Bologna, 1870.)

[3] Franco speaks of the " Maitres de bon aloi qu'il faut distinguer des periodeutes charlatans."   The more respectable of these peripatetics seem to have confined themselves to one country or district (*vide* note, p. 73).

operation gained both in method and in skill;
though as such a family depended for its reputation
on the possession of secrets real or supposed, our
records of their methods are few and insufficient.
At this time no surgeon graduate, not even Paré,
as I have said, dared to meddle with the operation.
The method of Celsus was with the finger in the
rectum to cut the perinæum transversely on the
stone without a director, and to hook the stone
forwards; for this purpose John of Gaddesden used
forceps. But such a blind method could not
answer well, except perhaps in children. The next
step, to pass a catheter or sound into the bladder, is
attributed to an unknown surgeon of Genoa; and
sounds and catheters of wax, tin, or silver were no
new things at the beginning of the sixteenth century.
Stricture of the urethra however in these centuries
was even commoner than stone. Franco, who did
more for the operation than any surgeon of the
sixteenth century, work indeed of permanent value,
took the lead in the lateral, and also in the high
operation—that is in opening the bladder for large
stones directly above the pubes, a method which
until his day was misliked. He pictured soft
sounds of lead, and many catheters, some with
stylets. Sanctus, a Neapolitan surgeon and pupil
of Vigo, fully described the median operation on
a channelled director, thitherto a secret. This
director, or " itinerarium," Collot got hold of, and
showed to Paré. Franco, who seems to have known
some Latin, probably got it directly from Sanctus'
Libellus aureus de lapide a vesica per incisionem

extrahendo, 1524; and as Franco's books were well
known in Paris (p. 76, note) Paré probably had this
higher authority in its favour.   Malgaigne confesses
that Paré was far from doing justice to his great
contemporary, who even in hare-lip was more
precise than Paré.   However literary property was
scarcely recognised in those days, and Franco in like
manner lifted much of his knowledge of syphilis
from the *Des bubons vénériens* of de Héry, to whom
neither Franco nor Paré seems to have been very
generous.   Paré defends plagiarism by the metaphor that every candle must be lighted from another
candle.   Fallopius was perhaps the first to recognise
literary honesty, at any rate in Medicine.

Unhappily in lithotomy the director fell into
disuse, and tearing and errant divisions of the parts
resumed their vogue.   Even the Collots were probably rough, bruising operators; and such was griev-
ously the case with the celebrated Frère Jacques,
who practised the lateral operation with prodigious
renown.   To him I am tempted to turn for a moment
in passing, although by his later date he lies out
of my proper limits.   Jacques Beaulieu, or Frère
Jacques, was born of poor parentage in Franche
Comté, in 1651.   He was a great friend to the poor;
but he was uncouth in manipulation, and his instruments were clumsy.   On his European celebrity he
received a friendly invitation to Paris from the
all-powerful Félix, and exhibited the lateral operation there; but things went ill with him, for out of
65 operations he had 25 deaths, and only 19 cures.
At that time at any rate he knew no anatomy; he

used to cut into the body of the bladder beyond
the prostate, so that urine was extravasated into
the cellular tissue of the pelvis; and he often
wounded neighbouring organs and blood-vessels.
At a later date, having learnt some anatomy,
improved his instruments, and introduced the staff,
he returned to Paris, when he is said to have
operated on 38 patients without a death.   By
care and skill Rau of Amsterdam, Cheselden, and
Hawkins reduced the mortality of Frère Jacques'
operation—in the hands of Cheselden to 7·5 per
cent.   Rau, according to John Bell, behaved in this
matter with duplicity towards Cheselden.

When Franco steps beyond his surgery he
becomes, as Guy in like manner, as blindly galenical
as the pure physicians.   He does not even suspect
that Galen had not to deal with lues.   In the
Middle Ages ophthalmic surgery also, in the hands
of barbers and wayfarers, had fallen into sad decay
and abuse.[1]   For eye surgery however the ancients
and the Arabs had done a good deal, and even
John XXI. something; in Bern and Lausanne an
illiterate practitioner like Franco would get access
to Celsus, and to Paul or Albucasis.   Franco practised his eye operations on animals, and on dead
bodies of men; and in the treatment of cataract is
full in his instructions and precautions.

I cannot make more than a passing reference to
the large and interesting subject of plastic opera-

---

[1] The best insight into the state of this department of surgery
in those days is to be had by perusing the treatise of Bartisch
Court barber, cutter for stone and oculist, in Dresden (1535-1606).
It contains good figures both of diseases and instruments.

tions which, after the times of Celsus and Paul, became the industry of specialists. The Brancas of Catania, who were celebrated nose restorers in the fifteenth century, seem to have got their knowledge from some stray MS. of Celsus. In the fifteenth century these operations had been many and important, probably because of judicial mutilations, free fighting, and syphilis. The material for regeneration was generally taken from one arm, which was bandaged to the face for some weeks. These operations fell into disuse till Tagliacozzi of Bologna rediscovered them two hundred years later. Paré and Fallopius rather ignorantly denounced them, and the clergy looked askance at such restorations, as a blasphemous invasion of the prerogatives of the Creator. After Tagliacozzi's burial, in the Convent of St. John the Baptist in Bologna, his cries in everlasting torment so disturbed the holy peace of the nuns that there was nothing for it but to howk his body out of its tomb and to restore it to unconsecrated earth. Even in 1742 that sublime body the Paris Faculty forbade such creative adventures altogether.

The very eminence of Ambroise Paré encourages, if it does not command me, to be content with few words of commemoration. If in some respects perhaps Paré may not be lifted far above his great Italian contemporaries, such as Carpi, Maggi, or Botallo, yet in a comprehensive judgment he surely stands alone in the surgery of the renaissance as an independent, original and inventive genius, and as a gentle, masterly and true man. Himself of humble origin he won for surgery in France a social place and respect it had never attained before. Born in 1517, he became a barber's apprentice in the Hôtel Dieu, whence he was called to join the campaign of Francis I. against Charles V. As he could not write a Latin thesis, his admission to St. Côme was of course opposed by the Faculty; but Paré stoutly and sagaciously declared that the vernacular[1] tongue was essential to the progress of Medicine; sagaciously, because the rise of the vernaculars from the fourteenth century onwards was as vital a factor in science as the formation of a latin medical prose had been.[2] Riolan the elder, who had taken part in the opposition to Paré, wrote a tract in 1577 with the following insolent title: *Ad impudentiam quorundam Chirurgorum qui medicis sequari et chirurgiam publicè profitere volunt pro dignitate veteri medicinae apologia philosophica.* To such inflated vanity the medieval " pure " physician lifted up not his mind only but his very soul. At this time, be it remembered, Paré was sixty years of age, and Surgeon to the King.

The first subject which comes into our thoughts with the name of Paré is that of the ligature of arteries; and you will scarcely desire me to pass

---

[1] Gale also wrote in the vernacular. The favour shown in the fifteenth century by the modish house of Este to the Italian vernacular (to Boiardo for example) gave a new impulse to its use in literature. The humanist, then as now, was fastidiously averse to vulgar progress. When, at Lorenzo's advice, Bernardo Rucellai invited Erasmus to answer his letters in Italian, Erasmus declined —lest he should spoil his style !

[2] One is tempted here to remark that Paré was testifying for his mother tongue seven centuries after Alfred, the pontiff of the vernaculars. On the formation of medical latin *vide* p. 25.

on without some discussion of it. I am often surprised to see, even to-day, the invention of the ligature attributed to Paré, whose surprise, if our journals have an astral shape, must be greater still, seeing that he himself, to justify an apparent innovation, refers the ligature to Galen. He says the ligature must have been taught him by the special favour of the sacred Deity, for he learned it not of his masters, nor of any other, neither had he found it to be used at any time by any. Only he had read in Galen there was no speedier remedy for stanching blood than to bind the vessels through which it flows. (Johnson's Edition, 1634.) The attribution is of course a legend. Malgaigne discreetly claims no more for Paré than the application of the ligature from wound-surgery to amputations; but I have implied already that even this claim goes beyond the truth of history. I must remind you once more that in all ages until the time of Paré the surgeons, for very intelligible reasons, shirked the larger amputations. Gersdorff indeed, a great surgeon of Strassburg of the previous generation, had rejected boiling oil and the cautery and, using only a styptic of hare's fur and white of egg, had performed two hundred of such amputations. He enclosed the stump in a bladder. The first picture of an amputation—it represents that of the leg just below the knee—is in Gersdorff's book (A.D. 1528). Yet it would be no great exaggeration to say that even to the time of Petit, who in the middle of the eighteenth century substituted the screw tourniquet for bandages

tightened with sticks and stones, amputation of
the larger limbs, save in gangrene, was avoided
as long as possible, and only too often longer than
that.   Celsus speaks of the ligature as an ordinary
method in wounds.[1]   From Oribasius we learn that
Archigenes of Apamea tied vessels even in amputation, after fixing a tight band at the root of the
limb.[2]   In the Middle Ages Yperman (p. 35) and
others—even Roger and Roland—knew the use
of the ligature, and Yperman indicates the method
as proper for arteries.   It seems probable that,
unless performed with modern nicety, secondary
hæmorrhage must have been frequent under ligature,
especially on the battlefield ;[3] indeed so late as 1773
Petit discarded the ligature, as Franco and Fabricius
had done.   Although Guy had endeavoured to
improve amputation, by drawing up the skin and
muscles, he never mentions ligature ; he used the
red-hot knife and styptics.   Paré however tells us
plainly enough that he undertook his experiments
with the ligature, and his improvement of this
means, because of the general experience of surgeons that the cautery, scalding oil, and styptics
such as rabbit's fur, aloes, and white of egg so
fouled the wound, and destroyed the flesh, as to set
up fever and to spoil the flaps which were then

[1] "Quod si illa (medicamenta) quoque profluvio vincuntur, venae
quae sanguinem fundunt apprehendae, circaque id quod ictum est,
duobus locis deligandae, intercidendaeque sunt, ut et in se ipsae
coëant, et nihilominus ora proclusa habeant."—Lib. v. c. 26, § 21.

[2] Paul on removal of tumours says "τὰ μὲν ἀγγεῖα διασφίξομεν."

[3] The best description of the ligature to be found in the seventeenth century is by Fallopius in the second volume of the Frank-
fort Edition of 1660, p. 210.

being designed and brought into practice. In contaminated wounds the cautery often acted no doubt as a purifier, as suppuration did (p. 30); but the means were indirect, precarious, and fraught with incidental mischief. It is a more intelligent service to a great man to point out how this detail and that of his invention were no mere incidents, but steps in a large reform of method; a reform which developed itself in Paré's hands on the introduction of firearms, whose ravages could not be covered up with galenisms.

If John of Vigo was not the first to mention, it seems he was the first to discuss the wounds of these new instruments of war. In a translation of Vigo's *Surgery* of 1514 is a chapter entitled *" Plaies faites de hacquebute, de bombardes et d'instruments semblables "* in which we read that Vigo shared the belief of the surgeons who first wrote of gunshot wounds, such as Brunswick and Gersdorff, that these wounds were envenomed burns; so that the chief aim of the surgeon should be to destroy the dead flesh and to neutralise the venom. To this end Vigo used the actual cautery, where possible; but for penetrating wounds the injection of boiling oil was more effective and convenient.[1] Berengar, Paracelsus, and Würtz did not accept the element of poison, but that of scorching only, and were content therefore with cooling methods; of their opinions, however, Paré had no knowledge

---

[1] I ought perhaps to say here that long before shot wounds were known boiling oil had been poured into any poisoned wound, as of venomous bites and the like, as the reader will readily discover, for instance, in Guy's chapters on wounds.

After a long verbal strife, the next step was made
by Maggi, who in a series of novel and interesting
experiments, published in 1551, discomfited Vigo
by firing balls at bags of gunpowder which did not
explode ; and arrows tipped with wax or sulphur,
which, however swiftly shot forth, respectively
neither melted nor ignited. Thus he disproved
the combustion hypothesis also. But to return
to Paré : the story goes that on the evening of an
engagement Paré administered the "first aid" of
boiling oil, as an antidote to the venom, to all
those injured by gunshot save one, for whom the
supply fell short. After tossing on his couch with
regret and apprehension, Paré rose betimes to see
this patient, in the hope no doubt of being enabled
to provide boiling oil for him also : but to his
amazement the unscalded limb was the best of the
bunch ; the patient had passed a fair night, his
wound was not angry, swollen or throbbing, as the
others were ; nor was he feverish. From this time
the receptive mind of Paré perceived that venom
and burn were figments both, and that a gunshot
wound was just a contusion or a comminution like
another. So severe however were the injuries of
gunshot, so frequently did these contusions become
septic, even in the greatest seigneurs, and so rife
the wound fever which, at the siege of Rouen,
Paré attributed in part only to a "malignant
atmosphere" and in part to putridity of the wounds,
that he determined to devote himself to the per-
fection of a more timely method of amputation.
It was as a part then of a great reform of method

that Paré was led to improve the ligature; his most orthodox patients proved not unwilling to forego boiling oil and the red-hot knife, and a successful early amputation of a smashed leg, at the siege of Damvilliers in 1552, placed his new method in safety.

Upon the many other contributions of Paré to surgery I cannot dwell; such, for example, as his ingenious method of detecting the course of bullets by placing the injured man in position as he was when he was struck—a plan first adopted by him in a consultation on the case of M. de Brissac. By this device Sylvius was so much pleased that he urged Paré to write his treatise *Des playes d'hacquebutes* (1546).[1] Sylvius (Jacques Delboe, or Sylvius the first) was the most erudite anatomist of the medical schools; yet Paré in his illiteracy had over him, as Palissy, whose demonstrations in his museum were attended by Paré, had over his learned audience, the ineffable advantage that when Hippocrates, Pliny and other great ancients came by translation within his reach, he read them in the unrefracted light of one practised in immediate contact with nature herself; and thus, without servility

---

[1] Vesalius, born three years before Paré, was also a pupil of Sylvius, who by the way was afterwards terrified to see what sort of a wildfowl he had hatched; but there was a great gulf between a lettered graduate and a barber's boy. Malgaigne reminds us that Vesalius' first anatomy and Paré's first tract on gunshot wounds were likewise published at the age of twenty-eight. How Paré pounced upon Vesalius' anatomy, how he used it "to verify his own experience," and how he prefixed to his *Surgery* a compendium of it, which during the next hundred years did more than the large and academic work of Vesalius himself to vulgarise the new anatomy, is too well known to be told again at large.

or prepossession, assimilated what he saw was masterly in them, as for example in the " Fractures and Luxations " of the Canon, upon which Paré drew largely.   But it was probably before he read Hippocrates that Paré described for the first time fracture of the neck of the femur.   He did not hesitate however to criticise Hippocrates, nor to differ frankly from him, or from Celsus, Paul, or Albucasis, if occasion required.   He writes " Il ne faut pas s'endormir sur le labeur des anciens comme s'ils avaient tout su ou tout dit."   As Guy was the last and greatest surgeon of the arabists, so Paré was the first and greatest of the renaissance ; Guy was the champion against medieval tyrants, Paré against the humanists and the Greek tradition.   Nor was Paré great on the positive side of progress only; he was no less resolute in confutation of fabulous lore.   If he believed in his puppy dog fat—and how could he resign a secret remedy which had cost him so many prayers !—he denounced, with an audacity which in our tepid and sceptical times we can scarcely appreciate, the bogus virtues of mummy and unicorn.   As great personages would marvel that he had not administered mummy in their lacerations,[1] Paré was aroused to indite his opinion of the stuff; and the King must have been annoyed to read farther that the horn of the unicorn at St. Denis, for which he had refused 100,000 crowns, was but an old woman's charm.

We parted from Henry of Mondeville carrying

[1] " Mummy," says Francis Bacon, " hath great force in staunching of blood, which may be ascribed to the mixture of balsams that are glutinous."

with us a pious and dignified sentiment; let us take leave of Paré with these words of his in our ears :—" You will have to render account not to the ancients but to God for your humanity and your skill." Was Paré the first modern surgeon to put humanity even before skill ? To us the barbarous practices of medieval surgery seem ferocious, yet we may reflect that in those violent days men's nerves were mercifully blunted, even, let us hope, the nerves of the patients.

In Germany, for all its meddlesomeness in Italy, Medicine, save in the debatable lands of Alsatia and Switzerland which drew some enlightenment from France, was in a barbarous condition. The manuscripts in Germany were few, and its universities, potent as they were to be in the emancipation of thought, were of later foundation than those of Italy. Germany had not even a St. Côme; and it would seem that, in the fourteenth century at any rate, there was no regular apprenticeship. Thus German surgery was grossly artisan, and therefore barbers and bathmen [1] flourished ex-

---

[1] The virtues of mineral waters and baths never lost the high repute attributed to them during the Roman Empire. I have before me a handsome thick folio in double columns *De Balneis*, published by Giunta in 1553, which is but one of those collections of treatises in the department of Medicine of which so many were published in Venice at and before this date. Some of my readers may remember Albert Durer's plate of a man's bath in a German town early in the sixteenth century. Becker (*loc. cit.*) includes bathmen among the practitioners, regular and irregular, of Hildesheim ["Aerzte und Wundärzte, Bader und Barbiere, Quacksalber, die Alexianerbrüder (a kind of sick club) Aerztinnen und Hebammen, und sogar—der Schinder !"]. Aachen was the fashionable spa in that district.

ceedingly.   Nevertheless even in the fifteenth
century, whither we may turn back for a moment,
some great surgeons had arisen in Germany; the
earliest of them who deserves remembrance was
Heinrich von Pfolspeundt—Pfalzpaint, in Bavaria,
south of Nuremberg—the manuscript of whose
Bunth-Ertzney had the fate of Yperman's treatise;
written in the middle of the fifteenth century, it fell
into oblivion until the nineteenth, when it was discovered in Breslau, and was published in 1868 by
Haeser and Middeldorpf.   Heinrich, like Paré and
many of the greater surgeons, was an army doctor
and saw much service; he was of noble family and
seems not only to have served but also to have
studied in Italy; yet he was unlettered, un-
instructed, and, as it would seem, knew only his
mother tongue.   As a wound surgeon ("Schäden
und Wunden") he left minor surgery to the
barbers, and the larger operative work to the
cutters ("Schneid-Aerzte"); on the other hand
he had learned "from a foreigner" the guild secret
of making new noses (p. 80).   His aversion from
the vulgar herniotomy was a rational aversion;
Pfolspeundt appears indeed to have been the first considerable surgeon to protest against the barbarities
of such specialists (*vide* p. 75).   In an appendix he
deals with some inward maladies.   Heinrich was no
anatomist, and in fractures and luxations a mere
empiric; moreover, in common with most or all
of his contemporaries, he was helpless in compound comminuted fracture.   Still he was a
shrewd, resourceful and not uninteresting person,

who divided wounds into fresh and foul; and
although, even in fresh wounds, he was a "suppu-
rator," and used turpentine and the like to promote
pus, yet he discarded tents, except for sinuses. For
hæmorrhage he does not mention the ligature; he
employed cold applications, and styptics on tampons.
In arrow wounds he had a large experience; he
was opposed to too much haste in extracting the
weapon, and to too early a use of the suture.
Of gunshot wounds he makes no mention. As
did the surgeons of all previous ages, he placed
much trust in "wound drinks," such as ptisan of
Artemisia and so forth. He devotes a section of
his book to the anæsthetic inhalation of Theodoric,
and recommends its use.[1]

In the history of the part of Germany in
European surgery we are apt, in the light of his
physical and chemical excursions and of his many-
sided character, to forget that Paracelsus (born
1491) was a surgeon, and no inconsiderable one.
Had this extraordinary man been endowed with a
little patience he would have been a leader in
wound surgery, though, like Würtz, and unlike
Gersdorff, he was not an operator. Paracelsus
pointed out not only the abuse of the suture by
the surgeons of the day,[2] but also that suppuration is bad healing. If left to herself, he declared,
nature heals wounds by a "natural balm," a phrase

[1] Guy of Chauliac tells us that sponges were impregnated with a
mixture of opium, henbane, hemlock, lettuce and other drugs and
dried in the sun. Before use a sponge was dipped in hot water,
and the patient then respired the vapours from it till he fell asleep.

[2] John of Vigo used the suture extensively, but always left an
exit for the pus (vide p. 9).

which Paré adopted (p. 31). In his *Grosse Wund-arznei* he says he began at the surgical because it is the most certain part of Medicine; and time after time he rebukes those who withdrew medicine from surgery. The unlearned, he says, speak of " surgical diseases," which is unreasonable, for Medicine (Artznei) is one (einerley). Called to the Chair of Medicine and Surgery in Basel,[1] he burnt Galen and Avicenna in the marketplace, lectured boldly in the vernacular, and declared reason based on experience of nature to be better than authority. Nature, he says, has her plan, and the physician's duty is to see fair play, and to keep the ring for her (pp. 42 and 97). Conrad Gesner (b. 1516), the naturalist and physician of Zurich, the friend of Caius,[2] in his wise way saved what was good in this revolt, and wrought at the ancillary sciences. To the dawn of natural science, however, the apostle of mystics was blind or waywardly averse. Rightly but too exclusively Paracelsus laid stress on function; as to every several function he gave its " Archaeus " so for him every disease was an entity, and every cure was to consist in an arcanum against the Archaeus. He had genius, but his experience was crude and precipitate.

Brunschwig (born 1497), the first of the great Alsatian surgeons, was, until the discovery of Heinrich of Pfolspeundt's manuscript (written thirty-

---

[1] It is interesting to remember that in the sixteenth century, Franco also was practising at Berne and Lausanne, and Würtz at Basel. Wittenberg was not founded till 1502.

[2] Whose *History of English Dogges* was composed for Gesner's *History of Animals.* Würtz may have met Caius (p. 94).

seven years before his own work), regarded as the
father of German surgery.   He was a barber, but
had received a good education in Bologna, Padua,
and Paris.   Like Würtz he was a wound surgeon and
bone-setter, and undertook no large operations save
those amputations which, in the case of the severest
injuries, became inevitable.   For Brunschwig, however, as later for Paré, gunshot wounds compelled
operative procedure more into prominence.   He
was indeed the first surgeon to enter upon the
surgery of gunshot wounds with any fulness or precision.   He too held that a gunshot wound was a
poisoned wound; and, to eliminate the poison by
free suppuration, used the medicated tents, or, in
case of through penetration, the setons, which were
to arouse the angry antagonism of Würtz.   If the
ball were out of reach in the body, he promoted
suppuration by poultices, turpentine and other
balsams; and seems to have hunted for the missile
with a kind of duck-billed speculum.   No wonder
erysipelas and phagedæna were rampant.   When
he was driven to amputate a large limb he bound
it above and below, drew up the skin before incision, and applied boiling oil or the cautery to the
stump.   With Heinrich he objected to anæsthesia
by opium, and used the narcotic inhalation of
Theodoric, which had some vogue all through the
Middle Ages (p. 90, note).   Like all the German
surgeons he wrote in the vernacular.

I would remind you again how large and various
was the experience of the battlefield, and how fertile
the blood of warriors in rearing good surgeons.

As Yperman and Paré, Gale and Wiseman, Maggi
and Botallo, so Brunschwig, Gersdorff and Würtz
won their spurs in Papal and Royal wars, as the
crusading surgeons had done from the Council of
Clermont to the fall of Acre.   Brunschwig, however, leaned heavily on Rhazes and Guy, and even
with gunshot surgery did not get very far ; a greater
reformer in this new military surgery in Germany was
Gersdorff, also an Alsatian, a man of great experience
and originality, and evidently a good mechanic.   As
did Paré and Wiseman, in amputation Gersdorff made
great use of the constricting band, to blunt the pain
as well as to check hæmorrhage.   He did not sear,
but used a styptic of his own, and covered the stump
with a bull's bladder.   In a more and more complete
retraction of the tissues before incision he made a
great improvement upon the old " sausage cut."   If
he probed gunshot wounds too eagerly, he did not
pour in boiling oil.   The works of both Brunschwig
and Gersdorff are illustrated, and not by drawings of
apparatus only; in both volumes are large and spirited
pictures.   In one of the illustrations of Brunschwig's
Surgery (Strassburg, 1497), for example, a man is
laid upon a couch with many and grievous wounds
upon him ; one of them being an ugly compound
fracture of the right leg.   A woman and two men
are deliberating on his case.   In Gersdorff's *Field-
book of Wound Surgery* (the Strassburg edition of
1528) is a lively scene of an amputation of the leg,
in which however it must be admitted that the cut
is shown very much after that of the " sausage."   In
another excellent woodcut two surgeons with some

mighty probe are digging for an arrowhead into the breast of a man seated on a three-legged stool. In the near distance an animated fight is in progress, and cannons and arquebuses, as well as spears, pikes and crossbows, are in full activity.

In Germany even of the sixteenth century there were no medical schools, not even of anatomy (p. 88). Thus Felix Würtz, if like Franco and Paré he had good fortune in escaping a scholastic education, was lucky also in the enjoyment of the more liberal education of Gesner's friendship. Gifted with an independent and penetrating mind, and aroused by the fiery disputes of Paracelsus, he is as fresh and racy as Henry of Mondeville had genius enough to be in spite of the schools. Like all his compatriots he wrote " *in sermone barbaro* "; and for its originality and conciseness Würtz's *Practica*, published in 1563, stands in a very small company. Had he known as much anatomy as Paré, his defect in which he bewails, he might have advanced in operative surgery and become as great a man ; for his clinical advances were both new and important. It is in the freshness and originality of his mind and in his freedom from scholastic convention, that he reminds us of Paré. Würtz protests against the kind of examinations for practice held in some cities, where candidates patter off cut and dried phrases like parrots, and apprentices " play upon the old fiddle the old tune continually." Surgery, he says, is a painful calling, and is not to be learned by sitting on a cushion at home. Who would order a picture of one who prates much of colours, but scarce knows how to hold a pencil ?   Würtz, being, as I have said, a wound surgeon, does not venture so far as Gersdorff in amputation, and the ligature he never mentions ; but he abhors barbarous blood staunchers, though in case of amputation of the thigh [1] hot irons must be at hand.   He has seen no reason to believe that bleeding is of use for " revulsion," nor that it " draws away humours from the head " ; it is a remedy to be used opportunely and discreetly.   Würtz is urgent on cleanliness ; clean hands, no hanging sleeves.   He protests against probing [2] and tenting, and dislikes poultice messes ; but as to suppuration, well, in spite of Paracelsus, it must be : he has never seen a severe wound heal without it.   As in any wound the virtue of coction is diminished, is not suppuration therefore necessary as a cleansing process ? (pp. 30 and 84). Still practice is better than conjecture, and if neither he nor Paré attacked suppuration in principle as Theodoric and Henry of Mondeville had done, Würtz, by setting his face against cataplasms and grease, made for progress.   Discreet as Paré and Würtz may themselves have been, yet the fidgety manœuvres, the probes and the plasters, the tents the salves and the setons, the handlings and the gropings, the meddlesome dressings, two or three a day, as the indications were incarnative, mundificative, maturative, cicatrisative, or consolidative, held on their fantastic and mischievous way.

[1] Perhaps the first definite mention of this grave operation ?

[2] " If there is more than one surgeon each of them must thrust his iron up and down in it, disturbing the healing balm, which should lie like a crystal on a clean wound."

Würtz's chief title to fame, a fame far less ripe
of course than that of Sydenham but, as it seems to
me, not unworthy to be remembered beside it, lies
in his clinical acumen; and especially in his development of the Hippocratic doctrine on wound in-
fections and their results; a doctrine which in
arabist tradition was embedded in a partial and
fragmentary way.   He publishes, as Paré did, and
as Salicet and Lanfranc had done, a large and
various collection of cases.   Watch, he says, and
learn to read any sign, be it never so mean; for
every day one may discover new secrets of nature.
Würtz divides wound fevers into three classes :—
First, those which set in with rigor, heat and sweating ; secondly, with pain in the wound followed by
repeated chilliness ; thirdly, with restlessness and
twitchings, the chills being less distinct.   He
says definitely that these disasters are due to
absorption of poisons from the wound.[1]   His description of diphtheria in throat or wound,—sometimes
first appearing in the one, sometimes in the other,—
when " prunella," as it is called in the only copy I
had at hand,[2] may be stripped off like a rag, is very
remarkable.   Yet on the curious German myth of
" joint-water " he is even more didactic and inex-
plicable than others of his compatriots of the period ;
a myth which that " ever angry " man Johann Lange
of Limberg demolished at last.   No surgeon of his day,
or before it, had given the attention which Würtz

---

[1] For a full account of these observations I refer the reader to
Billroth's *Historische Notizen über die Beurtheilung und Behandlung Schusswunden*, 1889.
[2] An English translation by A. L. Fox, London, 1656.

gave to conservative surgery. "Never, if you can help it, bereave a man of any part; for God's grace may be great upon it beyond the expectation of men." If this rule be more pious than definite, I may refer to his fuller details of splinting and bandaging joints, fingers, and other movable parts, in such positions that, if they must become stiff, they may give the least inconvenience.

Of the French Pox Würtz notes its peculiar influence on concurrent diseases and wounds; and that surgeons use mercury for it as indiscriminately as if mercury "were a saddle for any horse." He tells us not to thwart but to follow nature, "for she is as a strong river." He claimed truly that he had written no big book copied from those of his forerunners — for "naught will still be naught though practised for a thousand years"; that he had trimmed himself with no strange feathers, that he wrote only what he had made trial of, and that he had concealed nothing of what was known to him.[1]

In this period of German surgery it is convenient to mention that learned and skilful physician Wilhelm Fabry (or Schmidt) of Hilden near Cologne (1560 - 1634), usually known as Fabricius Hildanus; though he belongs in large part to the seventeenth century. He practised in Switzerland, was "Stadtarzt" of Bern, was associated with the Platters in Basel, and raised surgery in Germany to such honour and social con-

---

[1] I regret that Würtz's appendix on the management and cure of little children falls wholly outside my subject. It is full of wit, shrewd practice and common-sense.

sideration as to deserve the name of the German Paré. The several parts of his *Observationum et curationum chirurgicarum centuriae* were published at Basel from 1606 to 1646. With him we find not only that cases are published, as they were by his ablest predecessors (p. 33), but that his book consists of them; and we note, as in the Pentateuch of that other and greater Fabricius, " de Aquapendente," that we have entered upon a new kind of surgical literature. Fabry was far more than a " wound surgeon "; he operated boldly, and in the whole field of surgery. Like Vesalius he used the hot knife, which Paré had discarded; and in Gersdorff's fashion put the stump in a bull's bladder. Flaps were not adequately designed till a later date, but with a leather collar or compressor he carefully drew up the soft parts before dividing the bone, whereby also he prevented hæmorrhage. Thus he successfully amputated above the knee, but perhaps not—as his latest biographer alleges—for the first time (p. 95)? For hæmorrhage he sometimes cauterised, but sometimes he drew out the vessel with forceps and tied it with ligatures of flaxen thread. Another hundred years were to pass before the ligature became the general and predominant method. His examples of syphilis were a notable contribution to the history of this grievous and in those days terrible pestilence. He believed it to be transmissible on clothing and the like. For wounds Fabry favoured a simpler surgery, but he was no little of a galenist and refused to follow Würtz in the repudiation of pus. He cannot be ranked with the far-seeing men who once more advocated healing by first intention.   And in the third quarter of the nineteenth century, in my callow days as a physician, the apothecary of a large hospital showed me a row of amputations, with stumps pouring out pus in cataracts upon the cushions, and exclaimed—"That, sir, is what I like to see; nothing so wholesome in a wound as a good discharge of laudable pus."   As a university graduate,—for as universities were then we knew nothing of surgery,—I assented in superior ignorance.

England, if by England in the Middle Ages we mean no more than the Isles of Britain, made no progress in medieval or early renaissance Medicine. The Wars of the Roses may have been too savage for surgery.   It was the misfortune of England, by whose surgeons in the nineteenth century Medicine was to be regenerated, that until the seventeenth century her master surgeons were few and insignificant; before Wiseman indeed, it were hard to find one worthy to rival even the slender merits of Arderne and Gale.[1]   Oxford and Cambridge, as they took their origin, took their fashions from Paris; Linacre and Caius were strongly humanist in bent;[2]

[1] If Italy while mistress of the formative arts produced great surgeons, does the poverty of England in these arts illustrate its defects in surgery, until both arrived with Hogarth and Reynolds, Cheselden and Hunter.

[2] It is fair to add that Caius was more than a humanist.   He wrote an important treatise on the Sweating Sickness, and was a professed teacher of anatomy.   Dr. Venn says that Harvey pretty surely attended the dissections of Dr. Grimstone in Caius College.

and thus in England the division of the house of Medicine into surgery and physic became as deep and more abiding than in France; so deep and abiding that the evil of it is still at work among us.[1]

Arderne was probably a better surgeon than Gilbert, or John of Gaddesden; but he is little more than a name. Nor after Mondeville, Guy, Paré, Würtz, or Maggi, is it very interesting to peruse Thomas Gale (1507-1586 ?). From Gale's pages however we learn how deplorable was the state of military surgery even in the constructive time of Henry VIII. Tinkers, cobblers, sowgelders, are not the worst of the words he applies to the army doctors. So terrible were the deaths and tortures under their hands, that better men were demanded; and of these was Gale, who on arrival at Montreuil found the wounds dressed with filth fit only for horses' heels. Like Würtz and Paré, Gale wrote in the vernacular, and like them again seems to have been a high-minded and gentle person. His *Certaine Works of Chirurgerie* was published in London in 1563, a stout duodecimo in Black Letter with a few rude woodcuts.[2] To each of the four

---

[1] In the days of my graduation in my own University, since eminent in Surgery, we were not examined in Surgery. We were only called upon to produce a certificate of having attended a course of lectures on Surgery and Obstetric Medicine, certificates which I suppose I produced, though I have no remembrance of the lectures. In examination indeed Surgery was expressly excluded, for the requirement was "The medical treatment of surgical and obstetrical disease." During the time of my studentship at St. George's I believe I never entered a surgical ward. Happily when I settled at Leeds I was instructed in these matters under the second Wm. Hey and the two Teales.

[2] Copies are in the libraries of Cambridge University and Caius College.

parts of which it consists there was a separate
title.   The " *Wounds made by Gonneshot* " is the
third part, and here lies Gale's chief merit, that he
withstood " the gross error of Jerome Brunswicke
and John of Vigo, that they make the wound
venomous." [1]   For this independent opinion I
think he deserved mention by Haeser.   Gale is
wise also in advising that if a ball has so entered
the body that there is much difficulty in reaching
it, it be left there rather than "cause mortal
accidents" by the surgeon's ferreting after it.
Eleven soldiers shot in the body, and thus let
alone by him on service in 1544, did well.

For the rest Gale is sadly galenical,[2] and his
pages are stuffed with unguents and other receipts.
Like many of the elder surgeons he had a styptic
of his own, which he honestly publishes.   I regret
to say he was no " first intention " man, but would
put his salves even into green wounds, a surgery
Sir Thomas Browne was unwilling for his charity's

---

[1] The title runs thus :—An excellent treatise of wounds made
with gonneshot, in which is confuted both the grose errour of
Jerome Breunswicke, John Wiga, Alfonse Ferrius, and others : in
that they make the wounde venomous, which commeth through
the common powder and shotte : and also there is set out a perfect
and trewe method of curying these woundes, newly compiled and
published by Thomas Gale, Maister in Chirurgerie.   Printed at
London by Rowland Hall for Thomas Gale 1563.

[2] Galen, like Aristotle, was dressed as a counterfeit in distorted
and conventional forms.   In a dialogue prefixed to the volume,
a dialogue which in scene and temper and even in expression
is curiously like Isaak Walton, John Yates says he has read
" Theodoricus, Brunus, Lanfrancus, Rolandus, Rogerus, Bartilpalia,
Wilhelmus, Guido, Brunswicke and Vigo "—an excellent list.   Gale
replies " What part of Hippocrates, Galene, Avicenne, Paulus,
Rhasis, Albucasis, and Haliabbas have you rede ? thees be of greter
authoritie."

sake to disparage in the good Samaritan; though in this case the wine may have converted it into a less improper medicine. There is no resisting the truth that hitherto the land of Harvey, Sydenham and Wiseman had not done much for any part of Medicine.[1] The great Elizabethan glory shed little of its light upon our profession. Even in the seventeenth century Harvey was a maker of physiology rather than of Medicine, and in surgery Wiseman was a bridge of one plank between the Stuarts and the great eighteenth century school of Cheselden, Pott and Hunter.

Amid the English barbers of the fourteenth century some members took the name of Barber Surgeons,[2] and it was in their ranks rather than in the universities or the College of Physicians[3] that, as we have seen, surgery was likely to be advanced; in technical education indeed the London barbers were rather active. Moreover in England, as elsewhere, the post of King's Barber was one of much influence and profit. If we may judge by Holbein's picture, many of the leading barber surgeons were men of dignity and intelligence. Not a few of them, as in 1595 the College of Physicians com-

---

[1] To a little quarto by John Halle, published in 1565, with a portrait of the author, I may allude, but it seems to be no more than a translation of Lanfranc's *Chirurgia Parva*, with an appendix on the current anatomy, and an expostulation against the beastly abusers of chirurgery and physick.

[2] They were denoted as " Barbers exercising the faculty of surgery." There was an unincorporated and, in numbers at any rate, an insignificant body or guild of surgeons, not well disposed of course to the Barbers; and thus by divisions the cause of surgery was weakened.

[3] In the sixteenth century the London College of Physicians deliberately avoided its privileges in surgery.

plained, tried "the lenity and sufferance" of this body by practising some physic. The Barber Surgeons were incorporated by Charter in 1462, and thereby obtained in London power of examination, of suspension of practitioners whether home or foreign, and of inspection of drugs. Moreover towards the end of the fifteenth century, by a policy too enlightened to last long, a sort of conjoint board, with a more or less shadowy guild of surgeons, was established for these ends. Yet in the sixteenth century this promise and privilege faded; and "all the king's subjects having knowledge or experience of the nature of herbs whether obtained by regular study or by divine favour, recovered the right of ministration to any outward sore or wound according to their cunning." Indeed in 1540 the unincorporated company of surgeons was merged in the Barber Surgeons Guild, to which the power of licensing surgeons was restored; and the bodies of four malefactors a year were assigned to the Guild. In that year also my own Chair of Physic was founded, but unhappily without this valuable endowment.

Of Spanish surgery in the sixteenth century I know nothing of my own reading : Haeser speaks of it as progressive, both in the simplification of wound treatment, and of apparatus. Three Spanish surgeons of this century are said to have claims of priority for the method of healing by first intention ; namely, by cleansing, exclusion of the air, and the use of drying and "conglutinating" dressings. When such claims were made again in the seventeenth century the claimants were referred to these Spaniards. Into the justice of this cause I have made no inquiry, for I need not repeat to you that any such claims must be put very much farther back.

Time will not permit me to dwell upon renaissance surgery by any narration of the large advances of surgery in Italy during the latter half of the sixteenth century. I can dwell no more on Vesalius than to remind you that he was surgeon as well as anatomist; and, in common with his great contemporaries Fallopius, Ingrassias, and Fabricius, did much to reduce the use of the cautery and to improve the method in amputations. Biondo of Venice in the same period protested against the mistrust of water on wounds, and used free irrigation; as Humphry was doing in my student days, before Lister's discoveries. The names of Maggi and Botallo I have mentioned already. Maggi's work on gunshot wounds was published, on his death in 1552, at Bologna; thus really coinciding with if not anticipating Paré's opinions; moreover, as I have said, they were attained by the experimental method (p. 85). The edition I used for this essay forms a part of a collection of excellent surgical treatises in a handsome folio published at Zurich in 1555.[1] The introductory research into the nature of gunshot wounds (p. 85) is admirable; and if the rest of the work be less original and too much occupied by the "concoquentia et

[1] In the Library of the Royal College of Physicians, London.

pus moventia," it is well and forcibly written and
scholarly in form and completeness. A still greater
surgeon who had to thank the Popes, those stiff-
necked enemies of peace, for a familiarity with the
lacerations of war, was Botallo, whose treatise on
gunshot wounds, an excellent and exhaustive work
on wounds of the head, breast, abdomen, and limbs,
was published in 1560. This essay may be regarded
as some compensation for his bloodthirsty and mischievous tract on Venesection in the same volume.

Now during the periods I have surveyed what
were the clerks of inner medicine about ? Here you
will be on your guard against the sinister ways of
the man with a moral ; for it is my moral that physic
was sterile in proportion to its divorce from surgery :
yet, in the time allotted to me, if I may illustrate
this theorem I cannot prove it. Happily we have
Sydenham's summary of the matter, to Blackmore
who asked what book on medicine he should read ?
" *Don Quixote*," was the answer : as if to say,—
" contemplate medicine, that ponderous fantasy, in a
gentle, pathetic, and ironical spirit ; be tender with
it as human endeavour, yet recognise it for the
baseless and insubstantial fabric that it is." That
the life of surgery from the thirteenth to the sixteenth century was comparatively vigorous we have
just seen ; but it were an ungracious task to ramble
through physic only to illustrate its chimeras. A
perusal of the first 200 pages of the excellent
John Freind's *History* would suffice. I think no

historian will deny that in those ages medicine, in the narrower sense of this word, was a painted effigy — hollow, turgid and reactionary. Until we reach the first treatises on Epidemics, as for example Fracastoro [1] on syphilis and typhus, and the Spanish physicians on diphtheria (garotillo),[2] it is hard to discover in " pure medicine " any vitality, clinical or scientific, unless it lurked in the Aristophanic scepticism of Guy Patin, in the chemical therapeutics of the elusive Basil Valentine and of Paracelsus, or in the foggy platonism of Cardan. Even the staple of it was intimately entangled in astrology, alchemy, fantastical humoralism, urinoscopies and sphygmoscopies, and other dialectical puerilities. Pharmacy was, it is true, purged of some of its grossest, loathsomest, and foolishest ingredients; and the champions of mercury and antimony climbed over the dialectical fence under a deadly fire from Paris : but it was by surgery, then the laboratory of Medicine, especially by the large and manifold surgery of war, that medicine was regenerated ; and by such handicraft as that with which Harvey laid bare the secret of the circulation, and dealt the last blow to the crumbling carcase of galenism.[3]

[1] Fracastoro may be regarded as the founder of the doctrine of Infection. A collection of many treatises on syphilis was published at Venice in 1567, fol. It contains Maggi's treatise of 1550. Galen is quoted three or four times in each of these tracts as an authority on the French pox.

[2] Thus Dr. Payne says that the strong points of Gilbertus Anglicus were his account (evidently at first hand) of the plague ; and also of variola and morbilli.

[3] We know that Harvey was but too familiar with the battlefield ; and, if we do not know that he operated upon the wounded,

One episode of inner medicine, however, I will
select to serve as an example of the state of this
side of our craft, namely, the schism on the place
of venesection ; a schism which had a far-reaching
effect in the discomfiture of conventional galenism.
The heresy was as follows :—the Arabs, on purely
conjectural grounds, had always taught that
bleeding should be derivative, practised, that is,
on the side away from the lesion, or even in some
limb far away from it.   In the common case of
pleuro - pneumonia, for example, bleeding was
practised on the arm opposite to the side of the
pain.   Now Brissot, a learned Professor of Paris, and
one conversant with the Hippocratic treatises, proclaimed in 1514 that bleeding should be practised
on the same side as the disease ; in order, as he
said, to remove directly thence the fouled blood,
and to attract the good.   A strife ensued, of pro-
portions which to us seem incredible.   Parlia-
ment stretched out its arm to suppress Brissot, and
at length banished him ; but the war still raged, a
war against the arabists which surged even to the
foot of the throne of Charles V., who proclaimed
Brissot to be as infamous as Luther.   Clement
VII. himself joined in the fight ; and one far

we know that in times of peace he operated both as surgeon and
obstetrician.   Dr. Robert Willis in his *Life* of Harvey (Syd.
Soc. 1847) makes the amazing statement that surgery in the
seventeenth century "had not shown any good title to an independent existence.   The surgeon of those days was but the hand
or instrument of the physician . . . though Harvey it seems did
not feel himself degraded—(as Dr. Willis might have supposed ?)—
by taking up the knife or practising midwifery " (pp. xxvi.-xxvii.).
As Dr. Willis was librarian to the College of Surgeons all this may
be " writ sarcastic."

greater than Clement, namely Vesalius. It so
happened, however, that in the midst of the fray
a kinsman of the Emperor died of pleuro-pneumonia;
and the rumour grew that he had been bled in
Arab orthodoxy. Thus all was thrown into confusion; the judgments of Bologna and Clement
died on delivery, and, while many of Brissot's
followers proceeded to drop bleeding altogether,
Botallo and his school turned vampire. Servetus
was against the arabists, whose hair-splitting pulse
and urine lore was falling at last into discredit ;
and even pus itself got into some disgrace. At
length, towards the end of the century, after all
this clamour, it became generally admitted that
Hippocrates himself bled on the side of the disease.
Thus the orthodox who had disdained an intimate
occupation with nature as common and unclean,
and who augustly, confidently, and superciliously
had been entertaining heresy for centuries without knowing it, were put to confusion. When
the sticks are dry, when men's minds are pre-
pared for a revulsion of opinions, a small crisis
may have great issues; and so it was with this
bitter venesection controversy. We might suppose
indeed that when reigning creeds have to submit
to such rebuff they cannot last long ; yet, as it
is far easier to preach than to think, men clung
desperately then, as they cling still, even to the
very skirts of them.

No better example, though of a little later date,
of the stupifying effects of obsequious scholarship
can be offered than that of Cæsar Magati. Magati,

a Professor of Ferrara, was by no means a pedant or
a dry-as-dust.   He was a man of considerable parts,
who might have appealed more directly to a large
personal experience ; and had he relied upon himself would have been a far more interesting man
than he now appears.   Out of his own observation
and intelligence he contributed no little to the
simpler and cleaner treatment of wounds, a subject
on which he published—in Venice (1616)—a
handsome book ; too handsome indeed, for not
content with his own counsels and proofs, for which
his elegant Latin is almost too fine a garment,
he must needs display his learning, or cajole his
readers, by incessant quotations from the ancients.
Page after page, and many times upon a page, he
hides himself under authority, or adorns himself with
antique frippery.   Two or three chapters are occupied in an attempt by glosses to warp Hippocrates
and Galen towards his own opinions.   Thus even
in the seventeenth century this scholastic sequacity
still tormented the books, those especially which
issued from the universities.   How well Magati
could have spared this otiose labour may be perceived from such a passage as this, in protest against
the incessant interference of the galenists :—" The
more frequently a wound is opened up, the more
frequently it is disturbed (interturbatur'), and nature
is distracted from her proper office."   He protests
also against the prevalent notion that wounds may
be healed too soon, as even nowadays some of us
suppose of an eczema.   And not rarely he says
such wise things as this :—" Scientia est quae opus

facile reddit, ignorantia vero difficile "—would that an introduction of this maxim into the heads of statesmen of our own time could be added to the " triumphs " of modern surgery !

The physicians of the later sixteenth century who, as practitioners of internal medicine, can be readily named as profiting by the advances of the ancillary sciences are very few. Of them were Jean Fernel (1485-1558), Professor of Medicine in Paris, and the eminent follower of Vesalius, the Basel anatomist Felix Platter (1536-1614). Fernel was one of the early explorers of the seats of disease. He distinguished the causes from the processes, placing the diseases in the solid parts, and their causes in the blood ; symptoms he regarded as functional perversions. He endeavoured, as Broussais did some three centuries after him, to trace the specific fevers to definite local origins. Platter on the same lines achieved even more. These two physicians did much to establish or rather to restore " solid pathology," as opposed to the humoral. Vigorous antagonists of galenism on the same lines, though smaller men, were Giovanni Argenterio (1513-1572), and Laurent Joubert, the renowned and high-minded Chancellor of Montpellier, physician to Catherine of Medici. Joubert (1529-1583) laid much emphasis on natural causes, on physical laws, and on obedience to nature. But in this department of Medicine such men laboured in vain, except as champions of a new order. Their followers, such as Jerome Cardan, the dogmatist of " contraria contrariis," of whom Haller said " sapienter nemo quum sapit, dementior nullus ubi errat," bitten by neoplatonism, abandoned themselves to the building of card houses ("speculative Prunkgebäude" as some one has put it), and were lost to Medicine and to science.

With the sixteenth century my survey must end : from this time Medicine entered upon a new life ; upon a new surgery founded on a new anatomy, and on a new physiology of the circulation of the blood and lymph.   These sciences, thus initiated, not only served surgery directly, but indirectly also, by the pervading influence of the new accuracy of observation and the enlargement of the field of induction, modified the traditional medicine of physicians unversed in methods of research, as we perceive in the objective clinical medicine of Sydenham, who was no ardent friend of the ancillary sciences, and of Boerhaave.   Physiologists tell us that destruction is easy, construction difficult ; but in the history of medical dogma this truth finds little illustration.   So impatient is the speculative intellect of the yoke of inductive research, so tenacious is it of its liberty of prophesying, that no sooner did Harvey, by revealing the mechanics of the circulation, sap the doctrines of the schools, than some physicians instantly set to work to run up a scheme of iatro-physics ; others to build a system of iatro-chemics, but upon Von Helmont rather than upon Willis and Mayow, while Hoffmann and his school resuscitated the *strictum* and *laxum* syllogisms of the Greek Methodists.

Fortunately for the seventeenth century those

busy schoolmasters, the fingers, were making their
way into medicine by other than surgical routes;
and by the physics of Galileo, by the anatomy of
Vesalius, by the experimental physiology of Harvey,
by the pathological scalpel of Morgagni, and by the
chemistry of Mayow, had built into its structure
some solider stuff.   Yet even in the seventeenth,
eighteenth and early nineteenth centuries English
physicians worked still aloof from such men as
Cheselden (the friend of Mead), Pott, Hunter, the
Bells, Hey, Astley Cooper, and Brodie; an alienation
made absolute by the establishment of the College of
Surgeons, separate from the College of Physicians,
in 1798, whereby the integration of Medicine in
unity was once more defeated, and is still prevented,
in spite of Lister, and of the masterly disciples of
Lister, who in the obscure diseases of the abdomen
and pelvis are doing no less intimate a service for
inward medicine than Avenbrugger and Laennec
had done in those of the chest.

In this sketch of the past, a sketch necessarily
indiscriminate but not, I trust, indiscreet, we have
seen that up to the time of Avicenna, medicine
was one and undivided; that surgery was regarded
truly, not as a department of disease, but as an
alternative treatment of any disease which the
physician could reach with his hands; that the
cleavage of Medicine, not by some natural and
essential divisions, but in arbitrary paltering to
false pride and conceit, let the blood run out of

both its moieties; that certain diseases thus cut
adrift, being nourished only on the wind, dried
into mummy or wasted in an atrophy, and that
such was medicine; while the diseases which were
on the side of the roots, if they lost their upper sap,
were fed from below, and that such was surgery.

Thus the physicians, who were cut off from the
life-giving earth, being filled with husks and dust,
became themselves stark and fantastic.   Broadly
speaking, pathology until the seventeenth century
was a factitious schedule, and medicine a farrago
of receipts, most of them nauseous, many of them
filthy; most of them directly mischievous, all of
them indirectly mischievous as tokens of a false
conception of therapy.   A few domestic simples,
such as the laxatives, were indispensable; for the
rest we are tempted to reflect that mankind might
have been happier and better if Dioscorides had
been strangled in his cradle.

This is the truth I have tried to get home to
you:—That in the truncation of medicine the
physician lost not only nor chiefly a potent means
of treatment, he lost thereby the inductive
method; he lost the only laboratory at his service;
he lost touch with facts; he deprived his brains
of the co-operation of the subtlest machine in the
world—the human hand, a machine which does far
more than manufacture, which returns its benefits
on the maker with usury, blessing both him that
takes and him that gives.

Pure thought, for its own sake, especially in
early life when the temptation to it is strong and

I

experience small, seems so disinterested, so aloof from crude utility and temptation of gain, that in the history of ideas the construction of speculative systems has played but too great a part, and occupied but too many minds of eminent capacity.   We are bound to assume that these speculations have served—and for aught we know may still serve— some good end.   It seems " unhistorical " to suppose that age after age men have busied themselves to build up these vast systems in idle exercise.   That nature is wasteful we know but too well; yet she is wasteful by the way, not in the main direction of her work.   If some of her seed falls on stony ground, if her rain falls on the just and on the unjust, yet in the main the sowing and the rain are fruitful and joyful.   Peradventure, in our modern conviction of the efficiency of the experimental method, we may be too ready to denounce methods alien to us but which, hard as it is for us to conceive, may yet play some lasting part in evolution.   In our own day and fashion may we not become even too analytical ; on our good side may we not be too exclusive ?   In the pale hue of inductive analysis, sick with too much deliberation, may we not lose resolution, overlook the concrete, and forget that if by any mode of generalisation we lose the individual in the type, and the concrete in the negations and eliminations of abstraction, we ourselves may fall by another route into the very error of the school-authors ?   If their search for entities was false, may there not be a sort of imposition in " laws " ?   When in the last analysis we attain to

unresolved axioms may we not err in calling ourselves " synthetic philosophers," in giving even to a
true residuum too solid a significance ?   An abstraction is an abstraction, whether it be a summation
of phenomena or a speculative vision ; and abstrac-
tions may carry us a long way from life, from nature,
and from action.

In the minds of academical teachers the notion
still survives that the theoretical or university form
and the practical or technical form of a profession
or other calling may not only be regarded separately,
and taught in some distinction—which may be true,
but in independence of each other ; nay, that the
intrusion of the technical quality by materialising
tends to degrade the purity or liberality of the
theoretical ; that indeed, if he have not to get his
daily bread, the high-minded student may do well
to let the shop severely alone.   Thus the university
is prone to make of education thought without
hands ; the technical school, hands without thought ;
each fighting shy of the other.   But if in a liberal
training the sciences must be taught whereby the
crafts are interpreted, economised, and developed,
no less do the crafts, by finding ever new problems
and tests for the sciences, inseminate and inform
the sciences, as in our day physics have been
informed and fertilised by the fine craft of such
men as Helmholtz, Cornu, and Stokes ; or biology
by that of Darwin, Virchow, Pasteur, and Lister.
At the commemoration of Stokes in Westminster
Abbey, Lord Kelvin honoured in him the " com-
bination of technical skill with intuition "; and

Lord Rayleigh admired in him " the reciprocity of accurate workmanship and instinctive genius "; appreciations no less true of the distinguished speakers themselves.   If it be true, as I have been told, that the University of Birmingham has a coal mine upon the premises, I anticipate that the craft of coal getting, by carrying practice into thought, will fortify the web of theory.

There exists no doubt the opposite danger of reducing education to the narrow ideas and stationary habits of the mere artisan.   By stereotyped methods the shopmaster who does not see beyond his nose may cramp the prentice ; and the prentice becomes shopmaster in his turn.   If in the feudal times, and times like them in this respect, manual craft was despised, and the whole reason of man was driven into the attenuated spray of abstract ingenuity, in other times or parts of society a heavy plod of manual habit has so thickened " the nimble spirits in the arteries " that man was little better than a beaver : on the one side matter, gross and blockish ; on the other, speculation vacuous of all touch of nature.   We need sorely the elevation, the breadth, the disinterestedness, the imagination which universities create and maintain ; but in universities we need also bridges in every parish between the provinces of craft and thought. Our purpose must be to obtain the blend of craft and thought which on the one hand delivers us from a creeping empiricism, on the other from exorbitant ratiocinations.   That for the progress and advantage of knowledge the polar activities of sense and thought should find a fair balance and an integration of function, is set forth judicially enough in modern philosophy, and is eminent in great examples of mankind.   Moreover, it is apprehended in the reciprocal tensions of faith and works, of hypothesis and experience, of science and craft, and so forth. In our controversies on theory and practice, on universities and technical schools, on grammar and apprenticeship, we see their opposite stresses.   The unison is far from being, as too often we suppose, one merely of wind and helm, it is one rather of wind and wing; it consists not in a mere obedience of hand to mind, but in some mutual implication, or generative conjugation of them.

"Nor soul helps flesh more now than flesh helps soul."

How these two functions should live in each other we see in the Fine Arts—in the swift confederacy of hand and mind in Dürer, Michael Angelo, Rembrandt, Velasquez, Watteau, Reynolds, Watts. Genoa, Florence, Venice, Japan never disdained the crafts.   The infinite delicacy of educated senses is almost more incredible than the compass of imagination.   When they unite in creation no shadow is too fleeting, no line too exquisite for their common engagement and mutual reinforcement.   The craft of Verrocchio becomes the magic of Leonardo da Vinci.   Leonardo and Michael Angelo, in genius perhaps the greatest craftsmen the world has seen, were as skilful to invent a water engine, to anatomise a plant, or to make a stone-cutter's saw, as to paint the lineaments of the soul, and to build the dome of St. Peter above the clouds of Christendom.

Solve the problem as hereafter we may, now we can take heed at least that energy shall not accumulate about one pole or the other. Our little children have a message to us if we would but hearken to them. Every moment they are translating action into thought and thought into action. Eye, ear, and hand are incessantly on the watch and in pursuit, gathering incessantly for the mind the forms of thought which as rapidly issue again in new activities. As we mature we gain indeed in power of restraint, but it is not that we shall cease to act, that the mind shall depose the hand; but that these variables shall issue in richer and richer functions. If we forget the hands, the cunning loom which wove our minds, if thrusting them into our pockets we turn our eyes inwards, will our minds still grow true? That by virtue of the apposable thumb, monkey became man is no metaphor; in its measure it is sober truth. The bane of our profession for the last millennium has been too much thinking; we have actually made it a point of honour to ignore the hands out of which we have grown, and in this false honour to forget that the end of life is action, and that only by action is action bred. While we profess to admire Bernard Palissy (whose lectures Paré attended) or Jean Goujon, the medieval masons or the medieval goldsmiths, we act nevertheless as if fine arts only are honourable, and mechanical arts servile ; whereby we blind ourselves to the common laws of growth, which, knowing no such distinctions, deal out barrenness to those who make them.   We begin even with our children to wean them from the life of imaginative eyes and of thoughtful fingers ; and, instead of teaching them to rise from simple crafts to practical crafts, to scientific crafts, or to lovely crafts, and thus to pursue the mean of nature herself, we teach them the insolence that, except in sports, the mind should drop the acquaintance of the hands.

Shall we wonder then that in this generation bold men call English people stupid ; all stupid save those few men of genius or rich talent who, like Gilbert, Harvey, or Darwin, were great enough to be true to eye and hand, and to breed great conceptions by their intimate coition with the mind ?   Shall we wonder then that Medicine fell into sterility when by most unnatural bonds surgery, her scientific arm, was tied behind her, when she was too squeamish for raw truth, when she turned her sight inwards from lusty nature to formulas ?   Shall we wonder that even in the eighteenth century, when Medicine had begun tardily to occupy herself in the crafts of pathology and chemistry, one visionary after another, striding in long procession athwart the barren wilderness of physic, still wasted his generation in fastidious evasion of the things that happen, and in vain pursuit of vacuous unities ! Happily, if to the high stomachs of our medieval forefathers surgical dabblings were common and unclean, still there remained some eyes curious enough and some fingers dexterous enough to carry

the art back to the skill of Hippocrates and forward
to the skill of Lister ; and by the mouths of barbers
and cutters, rather than of the pharisees of the
colleges, Medicine breathed her lowly message to
her children.

WE are requested by the Congress of Arts and Science of St. Louis, 1904, to append brief lists of the more important works on our respective subjects. The chief part of my Address was founded upon a study —virtually in all cases—of the original works of the ancient writers themselves, and upon a number of short monographs and other articles—many of them in periodicals—the titles and references of which it would be difficult now to collect; and the list would be a long one. I append a list of the more comprehensive works to which I am indebted :—

HAESER.—*Gesch. der Medicin.* 1875-81.
PUSCHMANN.—*Handbuch d. Gesch. d. Medizin,* 2 vols. Jena, 1902-3.
DAREMBERG.—*Hist. des sciences médicales.* Paris, 1870.
Abhl. zur Gesch. d. Medicin,[1] Ed. Magnus. Breslau, 1902 *et seq.*
HIPPOCRATIS.—*Op.,* Ed. Littré, 10 vols. Paris, 1839-61.
PÉTREQUIN.—*Chirurgie d'Hippocrate,* 2 vols. Paris, 1877.
CELSE.—*Traité de Médicin,* Ed. Védrènes. Paris, 1876.
GALEN, Ed. Daremberg (two vols. only published). Paris, 1854-56.
Oribase, Oeuvres d', Ed. Bussemaker et Daremberg, 5 vols. Paris, 1851-76.
PAULUS AEGINETA, Ed. Adams, 3 vols. Syd. Soc., 1845-47.
SALICET, GUILL. DE.—*Chirurgie,* Ed. Pifteau. Toulouse, 1898.
MONDEVILLE, MAÎTRE HENRI DE.—*La Chirurgie* (Soc. anc. textes Fr.), 2 vols. 1897-98. *Ibid.,* Ed. Nicaise. Paris, 1893.

---

[1] The tract on the history of Antiseptic Surgery in this series was issued after my Address was delivered, and I have not yet had time to read it.

GUY DE CHAULIAC.—*La 'Grande Chirurgie*, Ed. Nicaise.   Paris, 1890.

Yperman, Chirurgie de Maître, Ed. Broeckz.   Anvers, 1868.

BILLROTH.—*Historische Notizen über die Beurtheilung und Behandlung Schusswunden.*   1889.

FERRARI.—*Une Chaire de Médicine au XV. siècle.*   Paris, 1899.

FRANCO, PIERRE.—*Chirurgie*, Ed. Nicaise.   Paris, 1895.

PARÉ, AMBROISE.—*Œuvres*, par Malgaigne, 3 vols.   Paris, 1840-41.
Ibid., par L. Paulmier.   Paris, 1887.

Annals of the Barber-Surgeons of London.   1890.

ALEZAIS.—*Chirurgiens et Barbiers de Marseille.*   1901.

INDEX

THE END

R
131
A57
1978

R
131
.A57

1978